PERMANENT

WEIGHT LOSS SOLUTIONS

By John J. Finley

PERMANENT

WEIGHT LOSS SOLUTIONS

Guaranteed To Work

Increase Your Financial Net-Worth and Employers'

Profitability by Staying Healthy & Fit

by John J. Finley

www.pwlsolutions.com

http://pwlsolutions.wordpress.com

CONTENTS

.

MISSION STATEMENT

Our mission is to teach behavior modification techniques that help inspire people to pursue healthier lifestyle habits. Thank you for your recent purchase of this book, Permanent Weight Loss Solutions. I hope you enjoy reading this book as much as I have enjoyed writing it for you. The behavior modification techniques I have outlined in this book are the same ones I have practiced for almost 30 years. These techniques are so effective they will transform your life forever. Trust me: I know. They transformed me from a military "diet private" into a "weight loss expert," and my life has never been the same since. In fact, you can start losing weight while reading this book by following the weight loss plan outlined in Chapter 12. By the time you finish, I guarantee you will be thoroughly impressed. You must remember, you didn't gain weight overnight, so don't be too anxious and expect to lose it all at once. According to weight loss experts, the slower you lose weight the longer you are likely to keep it off. Since these same experts all agree that diets are ineffective solutions to long-term permanent weight loss, this book focuses more on behavior modification techniques, which have been scientifically proven to be more effective than any other weight loss method. Take control of your life, health, and wealth and start losing weight today. While global warming is an important issue, global obesity is just as important, if not more so.

Yours Truly,

Weight Loss Expert John J. Finley.

Disclaimer

The information provided in this book is offered as an educational and reference volume only. It is not intended to take the place of medical advice from your physician. If you are currently under the care of a doctor, it is advised that you consult your doctor before implementing any of the programs mentioned in this book. Permanent Weight-loss Solutions is intended to be used as a stand-alone preventive tool or in conjunction with other weight loss aids. The advice given is for informational purposes only and has been constructed to teach behavior modification techniques that relate specifically to permanent weight loss. These techniques are designed to help facilitate long-term weight loss results. This book is intended to help motivate you into making a conscious decision to eat healthier and make exercise a part of your daily routine. Any information acted upon in this book you commence at your own risk. The information in this book is not intended to diagnose, treat, cure, or prevent any disease. The author and companies mentioned in this book present this information for educational purposes only. Additionally, the bookstores, publishers, and distributors also present this information for educational purposes only. I will not be making any attempt to prescribe a diagnosis or medical treatment. The information in this book is only my opinion, and is based on my personal experience and research.

MY PERSONAL EXPERIENCE

CHAPTER I

$\mathcal{A}$s I look back some 40 years, I can vividly remember my insatiable passion for food. I once asked my mom if there would be any food in heaven, because I had no intentions on going there unless she could assure me there would. On another occasion, after my cousin passed away, I remember everyone standing around crying. I got upset and started crying too, but not because she had just died. I was crying because I was hungry and no one would stop crying long enough to fix me something to eat. I remember arriving early to school each morning and heading straight for the cafeteria, where after eating my own food, I would ask the other children for the leftovers on their trays.

While serving in the United States Marine Corps and attending boot camp, I had the privilege of being assigned the task of anchorman for my platoon during a game of tug-of-war. I was singled out and deliberately placed at the end of the rope, where I was instructed to simply sit down. It became evident that the extra pounds I carried around came in handy as I helped my platoon win the event that day.

At family gatherings, my brothers and I were part of what was known as the "clean-up crew." This meant if anyone had leftover food on their plates, my brothers and I saw to it the leftovers never reached the trashcan. When my uncle wanted to restock his deep freezer with fresh groceries, he would call my mom and ask her to bring my brothers and me over to devour his old inventory. In my early youth it seems like every thought was food, food, food and more food every waking moment of every hour.

Today it is almost frightening to think that I was so habitually addicted to food. Back then it felt as though I was helplessly out of control with this compulsive addiction. No matter how much I resisted, I was allowing the allure of food to control me. The more I ate, the more I wanted to eat, sometimes to the point of becoming physically ill. In my adolescent years this compulsive

1

behavior didn't adversely affect me because I was active and still growing. As I got older things started to change, and my body started changing dramatically as well.

The fact that my mom and aunts were exceptional southern cooks didn't help this condition. My siblings and I had no idea what boxed, pre-packaged foods tasted like, and instead indulged in deliciously made from scratch home-cooked meals that tasted a lot better than the stuff served in restaurants and sold in grocery stores today. We ate macaroni and cheese prepared with real cheddar cheese, butter, eggs, and evaporated milk. My mom was well known for making the very best scrumptious desserts, like homemade cakes topped with real caramel icing made from scratch. People would pay her to bake cakes, peach cobblers, lemon meringue pies, and other great-tasting desserts. My aunt's sweet potato pies, baked turkey, and homemade dressings were very popular dishes as well. Another aunt was also known for making the best southern-style fried chicken and mouth-watering, mountain-towering pound cakes. Yet another aunt was good at making candied yams, hog-head-cheese, chicken and dumplings, and egg custard pies. These women didn't cut any corners when it came to the ingredients they used. It was real butter and vanilla flavoring, nothing pre-mixed or pre-packaged. Even the caramel icing for the cake was made by mixing together evaporated milk, sugar, and vanilla flavoring. These ingredients were brought to a boil and then simmered on low heat for several hours until they caramelized.

As you can clearly see, becoming addicted to these types of delectable, great-tasting foods was very easy, and trying to avoid them was next-to-impossible because they were served at every family gathering. As you can imagine, packing on the pounds came with ease, and it wasn't just me, but it seemed as if everyone around me was also growing in size. I remember going school shopping with my mom when I was little. Back then the only apparel sizes available to the general public were small, medium, or large, meaning the extra-large sizes commonly worn today were only available as special order items in stores and catalogues. In fact, the average person today is about 30 pounds heavier than he or she was just 40 years ago which explains why small sizes today rarely leave the clothing racks of most apparel stores.

In addition to myself, my brothers, sisters, aunts, uncles, cousins, and friends were all graduating up to the next clothing size. Almost all of them were also actively participating in some sort of newly discovered diet plan with very limited success. In fact, government research has revealed some very staggering and sobering statistics about many such diet plans:

Ninety-seven percent of all dieters fail and that most regain their original weight plus a few extra pounds within the first 5 years of dieting. This is incontrovertible proof that dieting isn't the real solution for losing weight or keeping it off permanently. If diets were truly effective, a new one wouldn't be introduced almost every month.

The true answer to a successful and permanent weight loss career involves four basic principles:

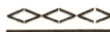

1) Behavior modification
2) Nutritional discipline
3) Dietary education
4) Incorporating routine exercises that are both fun and easy

By my late teens it had become abundantly clear that my uncontrollable passion for food had started taking its toll on my health and physique. The couple of pounds that I could have so easily have shed when I was younger, were starting to stick around and weren't budging. The clothes I normally wore didn't seem to fit the same anymore, even though I was dieting and exercising vigorously on a regular basis. These excessive pounds were beginning to adversely impact my health as I was diagnosed with hypertension and my weight had become embarrassing. I was on a newly discovered diet plan almost every month of the year. I tried all types of diet plans: salad, fat-free, sugar-free, dairy-free, carb-free, meat-free, cereal, fruit, and water diets. I even tried fasting, but that didn't last very long. Some of these diets had positive initial results, but the results were just temporary solutions without long-term impact.

One reason for this was none of these diets was feasibly practical or reasonably sustainable life-long solutions to my weight problem. I wasn't going to just eat cereal and fruits for the rest of my life. I would soon get bored eating salads three times a day. Fat-free diets are not good because the body requires a balance of the important essential fatty acids to help maintain optimal health. As much as I enjoyed eating, fasting was definitely out of the question. Simply drinking water would eventually become detrimental to my health. As my food addictions spiraled out of control so did my desperate search for a new diet plan to fix the problem. I had always been a stickler for being physically fit, but now I was starting to lose my physique. The harder I tried to stop this pending disaster the more pounds I was packing on. I was being transformed into someone I had never dreamed of or ever wanted to become.

In reality, I was my own worst enemy even though I didn't want to admit it. To me, food was the problem, so I attacked the food instead of attacking myself. It was too painful for me to deny myself the types of foods I enjoyed eating. I was living to eat instead of eating to live. I had no nutritional education as it related to proper food combining techniques and healthy lifestyle habits. My behavior to-ward food was unhealthy and needed an overhaul. Eventually, my unhealthy lifestyle and mentality took its toll.

The straw that finally broke the camel's back happened when I joined the United States Marine Corps. While in boot camp I received some very sobering and devastating news from my senior drill instructor. I was told that because of my excessive weight, I would not be allowed to graduate with my platoon and would have to spend some extra months in training. As much as I loved the Marine Corps, boot camp was another story, and I couldn't wait for it to be over. In order to graduate with my class I would have to shed almost 30 pounds in 8 weeks.

I was given the option of becoming what's known in the Corps as a "diet private" or keeping the pounds and extending my stay in boot camp. The fear of not graduating with my class that summer forced my hand. I decided that the prospect of spending even one extra day in boot camp was not an option for me. In the end I agreed to become a Marine Corps diet private. My new status meant I would have to drastically change the way I ate. I was restricted to eating only certain types of foods like fresh fruits, vegetables, salads, cereals and meats. All desserts, sugary sweets, and sweetened beverages were strictly off limits. One day, I got bored of just eating vegetables and decided to take a chance and cheat a little. Unfortunately, I didn't know I would be caught that day by my senior drill instructor. As fate would have it he just happened to be seated at a table near the end of the chow line.

While leaving the chow line, I impulsively grabbed a couple of items I fully knew were forbidden and off limits. When I walked passed my senior drill instructor, he called out my name and motioned for me to come over to his table. As I headed in his direction my heart started to sink into my shoes, as I nervously anticipated his reaction. He calmly asked what I was doing with forbidden delectable items on my tray. While still seated, he started shouting at me and violently kicked the tray out of my hands spilling food all over the floor. He scolded me and ordered me back to the beginning of the chow line where I had to start all over again. The chow line was designed so that as one platoon entered the mess hall to eat, another platoon entered in right behind it. This procedure expeditiously facilitated the feeding of many Marines in a timely manner. Each platoon was allowed a few minutes to sit down and eat. This meant that by the time I went back through the chow line, my platoon had already finished eating.

Though I didn't get the opportunity to eat lunch that day, I did graduate with my platoon. Moreover, my weight loss transformation was so dramatic and successful my own family didn't even recognize me when they came to visit one week before my graduation. In fact my mom, dad, siblings, and friends walked right passed me without recognizing who I was. I had to literally grab them by their arms and convince them I was the Marine recruit they had traveled so far to visit.

I hope you don't feel too sorry about my missed meal that day in the mess hall. Truth be told, it was the best thing that could have ever happened in my life. The Marine Corps taught me the self-discipline and motivation needed not only to lose weight, but to keep it off permanently. Those humiliating and embarrassing days I suffered through back then have enabled me to help countless individuals reach their personal weight loss goals, better their overall health, and improve their quality of life.

Were it not for my Marine Corps diet private experiences during boot camp, I probably wouldn't be alive today, or at best I would be in very poor health. The greatest personal benefit for me has been the fact that I haven't needed to use dieting, diet aids, or medical intervention to maintain my weight. Those experiences allowed me the opportunity to take a serious look at my eating habits and examine the psychology of my behavior toward food, nutrition, and fitness.

Since that time, I have maintained the same basic principles that I teach to others as they relate to permanent weight loss strategies:

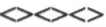

1) Always pay attention to what goes into your mouth.
2) Drink water as your primary source of hydration.
3) Incorporate routine exercises into your weight management and weight loss program.

In order to have a successful and long-term weight loss career, you must apply these three core principles. Over the years, I have received countless testimonials from various individuals who have successfully lost weight and kept it off while employing these principles. Although there are many diet products, weight loss centers, and newly discovered diet drugs, obesity has now become the number one global health threat. What separates this book from all the others is the fact that it doesn't teach you how to become a better dieter. As I mentioned earlier, according to the latest government statistics and visible evidence, dieting is ineffective in generating permanent and long-term weight loss success. Former Arkansas Governor Mike Huckabee, himself an inspiring weight loss success story, stated that he incorporated behavior modification techniques that literally saved his life. At the time, he was 100 pounds overweight and suffering with diabetes. He had tried diets and concluded that they didn't work; there was no magic weight loss cure.

Changing his lifestyle not only enabled him to lose over 100 pounds, but also helped to cure his diabetic condition. He stated he no longer needed to take diabetic medications and attributed the success of his improved health to the behavior modification techniques he had recently incorporated. There are no physiological differences between Mike Huckabee or you and I. He simply made the necessary changes and the positive results followed. I went through this same transformation more than 27 years ago, losing over 50 pounds and never gaining it back. This lifestyle approach has worked for countless individuals and it will work for you. The key to permanent weight management is not allowing your environment to dictate the type of lifestyle habits you choose to incorporate.

THE PERFECT OBESITY STORM

CHAPTER II

*O*n several occasions I tried to figure out which events over the past 70 years could be responsible for causing or greatly contributing to the current global obesity crisis. As I researched various theories, certain observations reverberated dramatically through my mind. I began to diligently study these events, and was overwhelmed by the evidence supporting my hypothesis.

I decided to group these events together into what I've termed "The Perfect Obesity Storm." This perfect storm has involved events that have taken place over the past half-century and have resulted in unintentional catastrophic complications such as obesity and obesity-related diseases like diabetes, heart disease, cancer, and myriad other health problems. It is also my deepest belief that this perfect storm has contributed to obesity now becoming the number one global health threat. With that said, I strongly believe that if we collectively work together to reverse this storm, the world will experience a precipitous decline in the escalating trend toward obesity and the prevention of almost 30 obesity-related diseases.

As I explain the events in this book, you too will be convinced that there is some validity to my observations. There is a term in the world of physics known as cause-and-effect; for every action, there is an equal and opposite negative or positive reaction. In other words if you indulge in poor eating habits and a sedentary lifestyle, you can expect to suffer poor health. However, if you do just the opposite you'll more than likely be a healthier person according to medical experts. Before I proceed any further, I want to explain a fact related to our human anatomy. The human body hasn't experienced any type of physical or physiological changes over the past 70 years. That could explain the current obesity epidemic. In fact, our bodies continue to function pretty much the same way for as long as human beings have existed. Our basic physiological need for water and salt has remained constant throughout time, as both of these elements are vitally important for our very existence. We continue to walk upright and consume food through our mouths, hear with our ears, see with our eyes, and smell through our noses. Since our bodies haven't changed much over time physical change can be excluded as contributing to the obesity epidemic.

The only other place to examine, then, is the environment in which we live. As we begin to examine and piece together these environmental changes, things seem to fall in place rather clearly.

Today America is one of the wealthiest nations in the world, spends the most on health care, and sadly ranks just 42nd in life expectancy globally; obesity has been implicated as one of the main reasons for this. More importantly, obesity is fast becoming an epidemic of global proportions and poses one of the greatest threats to human health and well-being in the 21st century. The World Health Organization has stated that obesity is a disease of pandemic proportions, and that it threatens the developed and developing world alike. Some of the heaviest people on the face of the earth live in America, where almost two-thirds of the population is overweight. Included in this number are roughly 59 million Americans who are considered obese, putting themselves at risk for developing heart disease, diabetes, hypertension, and various forms of cancer. It is predicted that by the year 2017, obesity will become the number one preventable cause of death in the U.S. Again, these are problems that can be averted if we collectively take immediate action to address and reverse this perfect storm.

In order to properly analyze this storm, we must first consider certain internal and external environmental changes that have evolved separately before we can tie everything together. The unhealthy external environmental events that have converged are as follows:

First on the list is our societal switch about 70 years ago from eating nutrient-rich whole grain-based foods to consuming mainly industrialized, refined, nutrient-depleted commercialized food products. When they are processed, these foods are bleached and stripped of naturally occurring life-sustaining vitamins, minerals, fibers, digestive enzymes, and disease-fighting antioxidants and phytonutrients.

Next on the list was the nascent introduction of fast food and junk food products. In my opinion these are far worse for our health because they contain potentially harmful substances that are added to make a little product stretch a long way or stay fresher longer. Ingredients such as ammonium-hydroxide and other genetically modified food additives.

Third on the list are hydrogenated or trans fatty acids. Trans fats are fat molecules artificially manipulated and transformed by humans into a highly toxic substance that adversely impacts every biological function in the body. With the introduction of trans fats, our primary sources of omega-3 essential fatty acids were replaced with the introduction of hydrogenated or trans fatty oils. Trans fats are so deadly to human health, many states have banned their use in food products sold to consumers. Dr. Walter Willett, chairman of the Department of Nutrition at the Harvard University School of Public Health, praised New York health officials for banning trans fats, which he said could save lives. He argued that artificial trans fats are very toxic, and they almost surely cause tens of thousands of premature deaths each year. Dr. Willet added his belief that the federal government should have banned trans fats a long time ago.

By the end of World War II, most of the country consumed trans fats because they were touted as a healthy replacement to saturated fats in our diets, which at the time were derived mostly from animal and dairy products. Also, as the war progressed the use of products made from trans fats such as margarine increased sharply as butter was being rationed to soldiers fighting the war overseas. Unlike saturated fats that contain tiny amounts of essential fatty acids, trans fats contain virtually none of the fatty acids the body requires to help maintain optimal health. Essential fatty acids are vital to every metabolic function in our bodies.

It is believed that trans fats interfere with the body's ability to ingest and utilize the healthy fats in our diets. Today trans fats are principally made out of non-fermented soybean oil, which depresses the thyroid, resulting in lower energy levels. This makes a person feel less motivated to exercise, which ultimately results in unwanted weight gain. Many medical experts strongly believe that hydrogenated oils have greatly contributed to the epidemic levels of obesity and related diseases that developing nations are now experiencing. Fourth on the list of unhealthy external environmental events is the excessive consumption of refined sugar, salt and artificial sweeteners. At the turn of the century, the average person consumed just 3.5 pounds of sugar annually as compared to an astonishing 140 pound annual average consumption rate today.

Fifth would be the overuse of antibiotics, and second hand antibiotic exposure from animal and dairy products, which destroys our friendly intestinal bacteria. Added to this are high levels of growth hormones and steroids in our food supply. In addition, there has been an unprecedented rise and expansion in the use of prescription and over-the-counter medications.

And finally, number six, many people simply do not drink water anymore. Instead, people drink unhealthy, highly-sweetened carbonated beverages and fruit juices, such as those that accompany high calorie, nutrient-deficient, super-sized meals offered by the fast food industry.

Even our children are raised on baby formula, which lacks all of the healthy life-building and protective benefits that can only be found in human breast milk. Recent studies suggest that children weaned on baby formula are more likely to become overweight as adolescents than their peers weaned on mother's breast milk. It is the sum total of these external environmental events that, over time, have negatively altered and impacted our body's internal environment, causing it to become dangerously unbalanced.

Today, we suffer with constantly elevated insulin levels, which trigger our bodies to store more fat. Our intestinal micro-flora (bacteria), which are responsible for keeping us healthy, are overgrown with damaging, unfriendly, and hostile bacteria. These hostile bacteria prevent proper digestion, assimilation, and elimination of the foods we eat. Hostile bacteria have a voracious appetite and require more than six-and-a-half times the same amount of glucose for fuel as our normal, friendly bacteria.

You've probably had the experience that upon finishing a fairly good-sized meal, soon afterwards you were still hungry. Don't feel bad; it wasn't your fault. You're feeding trillions of uninvited guests (unhealthy bacteria). It is believed this condition could possibly be responsible for generating as much as 10 to 15 pounds of excess body weight. The adverse relationship between intestinal dysbiosis and unwanted weight gain due to increased sugar and starchy cravings will be further explained in chapter 3.

Most of the foods we eat today are non-water soluble, absent of fiber, and highly processed with sodium, which causes us to consume more liquids than we would normally drink. The more than 80 balanced minerals that naturally occur in real salt have been stripped away, leaving behind a deadly combination of sodium and chlorine. When this poison enters our bodies, it forces our cells into survival mode by entombing themselves in excess water for protection, resulting in fluid retention and extra body weight.

Most of the moisture in our food is removed through overcooking and exposure to excessively high temperatures. With the removal of moisture, our foods also become less hydrated which also increases the need for additional fluid intake. Highly processed foods interfere with the body's natural ability to produce the proper appetite suppression and hunger-regulating hormones. If these hormones aren't constantly balanced, one will not be able to control his or her appetite, and habitually resort to overeating. Furthermore, certain types of calories consumed, especially those in the form of high fructose corn syrup, can actually cause a person to gain weight even though his or her overall daily caloric intake is minimal. For some reason not yet known to scientists, the body processes this manipulated sweetener differently than ordinary sugar. Unfortunately, today just about everything sold in restaurants and grocery stores contains this unhealthy garbage. It's used in baked goods, lunch meats, soft drinks, jellies, desserts, bacon, breads, crackers, fruit drinks, syrups, and many other items. Even food products labeled as "all natural" can contain high fructose corn syrup as a sweetening agent. In fact, because this sweetener is very cheap to manufacture, it's a food processor's dream ingredient, saving them lots of money, which keeps shareholders happy while keeping us fat.

Meanwhile, high fructose corn syrup has greatly contributed to the obesity crisis since its introduction to our food supply almost 30 years ago. While glucose is readily metabolized by every cell in the body, fructose must first be metabolized by the liver. The average person unknowingly consumes massive amounts of fructose every year. In lab tests, animals given large amounts of fructose developed a condition known as fatty liver disease or Nonalcoholic Steatohepatitis. This disease, known as NASH, is similar in nature to cirrhosis of the liver, which is caused by excessive alcohol consumption. With NASH, the liver becomes overly saturated with fatty deposits and cannot function properly. It actually turns into a great big sack of fat.

The liver is responsible for burning and distributing fat evenly throughout the body. Although many of us consider our heart and brain to be the most important organs, you'd die in roughly 24 hours if your liver stopped functioning. It has the vital task of transforming food into nutrients, maintaining fat metabolism and distribution, removing harmful substances and preventing certain environmental chemicals we're exposed to from becoming cancerous in our bodies. Therefore, if the liver is bogged down with this excess fat and unable to function properly, gaining unwanted weight becomes inevitable.

Most of the commercially-processed foods available today contain a combination of anywhere from two to five different types of sweeteners. For example, you may pick up one item that contains sugar, corn syrup, high fructose corn syrup, and dextrose. This one product has four sweeteners, with high fructose corn syrup and sugar as the main ingredients. Now combine this single item with other highly-refined starchy food items that lack plant-based fiber (which slows the rate at which glucose enters the blood stream). By slowing the rate at which glucose enters the blood, blood sugar levels are kept stable, preventing excessive insulin from triggering fat storage. These items are normally eaten with a high-fat, high-protein protein sandwich or deep fried meat product. All of this is then topped off with a triple-sized 42-ounce serving of your favorite beverage, which also contains huge amounts of high fructose corn syrup or some other artificial sweetener.

Every day, millions of people happily consume these types of meals, with most being brainwashed into actually believing it's nutritious. This example reveals how easy it is for dangerous amounts of sugar to quickly accumulate in the body after consuming just one meal. Again, the body is designed to tolerate small amounts of sugar for short periods of time. The problem is further complicated by the fact that most people do not exercise regularly, allowing dangerous amounts of sugar to build up in their bodies.

It was once believed that replacing refined sugar in our diets with artificial sweeteners would actually be better for our health and help us manage our weight. The switch to artificial sweeteners was made almost 30 years ago, and today people are sicker and fatter than ever. These are some of the reasons some nutritional experts are now advocating a return to refined sugar while staying away from artificial sweeteners. As glucose is recycled through the body, it becomes poisonous and can no longer be used as a viable source of energy. A healthy functioning liver would normally try to convert part of this toxic waste into a salvageable fuel source. Because of all the toxic substances the liver has to process (like antibiotics found in most meats and dairy products), it could easily become over-worked, and possibly over time eventually break down under such stressful conditions. With the liver out of action, every other normal bodily function is thrown completely out of kilter.

Yes, I believe the perfect obesity storm, comprised of various external and internal environmental events that appeared on the horizon some 70 years ago, has finally converged within our bodies, resulting in epidemic levels of obesity and chronic degenerative diseases. Since the inception of the "perfect obesity storm," the rates of cancer, heart disease, diabetes, hypertension and obesity have all dramatically increased. However, if we look back just 100 years, before the storm clouds started gathering together, we will discover a very interesting picture. We will see that the external and internal environmental landscape previously mentioned for causing the perfect storm was in reverse order.

The foods people consumed at the turn of the century were full of natural nutrients and free of growth hormones, antibiotics, pesticides, and chemical fertilizers. Back then, the number one cause of death in the United States was not obesity-related diseases but infectious diseases. In fact, it was not a common sight to see morbidly obese people walking around like today. The only things that have dramatically changed over the past 100 years are the condition of our foods, our primary sources of hydration, and our level of physical activity. Our food is imbalanced and highly refined, which keeps our bodies unbalanced. Consuming these foods while over-hydrating with sugary beverages keeps insulin levels in the body constantly elevated causing extra weight gain.

Finally, we don't get out and exercise on a consistent basis; if we did so, it could lessen the impact of being constantly exposed to elevated insulin levels. The unprecedented explosion in body weight has impacted not only us humans, but everything in our environment as well. Today, our domesticated pets are just as obese as we are.

Recently the FDA approved a weight loss pill called Slentrol available for the management of canine obesity. Yes, it appears as though man's best friend has been adversely impacted and handicapped by this perfect obesity storm. At the current rate, obesity will soon be the norm, as well as the leading preventable cause of death in the United States, outpacing both heart disease and cancer.

The number of overweight and obese people is truly staggering, particularly amongst our young children. Whoever gets caught in this perfect obesity storm's insidious and destructive path becomes a victim; it affects young and old, rich and poor, all races and creeds. If we are going to reverse the direction of this now pending global obesity pandemic, we must travel headlong into the eye of the storm and dissect the root causes of its origin. We must travel back through time before the obesity problem got into full swing.

Fortunately, we won't have to travel that far, just 70 years or so, when the word "obesity" was virtually unheard of. It was right around this same time that the population as a whole started changing its dietary habits and became more sedentary. Farmers have known for thousands of years that feeding an animal grains can make them fatter, as long as they are not allowed to run around too much. As it turns out, this applies to humans as well. It is interesting to note that as rare as obesity was back then, so were conditions like diabetes, heart disease, and cancer. This means that, in one way or another, these diseases are all inextricably tied together. It is this relationship that makes tackling the obesity epidemic an even higher priority.

Fortunately, reversing the perfect storm is not as difficult as one may think. According to the experts, obesity is neither a medical nor a scientific problem, but rather a behavioral one. In other words, resolving obesity is not academic; it's common sense. With that said, the most logical way to attack the problem is to approach it with behavior modification techniques. These techniques should cover what I call the "Seven Key Steps" to permanent weight loss management. When these key areas of health and nutrition are mastered, the perfect storm will be put to rest and vanquished once and for all. These key areas are proper nutrition, hydration, physical activity, digestion, assimilation, elimination and a balanced intestinal flora ratio.

Proper nutrition involves eating foods that have been minimally processed and offer a rich source of vitamins, minerals, natural fiber, digestive enzymes, antioxidants and phytonutrients.

Proper hydration is simply making water 90% of your total daily fluid intake, with the remaining 10% being sweetened beverages. These sweetened beverages should be consumed between 30 minutes and 1 hour before working out.

Physical activity includes routine exercises lasting no less than 20 minutes in duration. They should incorporate both strength training and low-impact aerobic activities performed four or more times per week.

Proper digestion involves good eating habits that allow the body to naturally produce protective hormones that prevent diseases and overeating.

Assimilation involves keeping our intestines constantly cleansed and in good working condition so that nutrients from the foods we eat can be efficiently absorbed.

Elimination involves the amount of time it takes food to be processed out of the body. The quicker food is broken down and eliminated from your body, the easier it will be to lose and manage your weight.

Balanced Flora having a proper balance ratio of healthy and unhealthy intestinal bacteria (Flora), could help shed excess pounds and greatly curb hunger and sugar cravings.

These seven key steps are the foundation and building blocks to good health and optimum weight management. With these seven areas in proper working order, you will effortlessly overcome the battle of the bulge. No longer will you have to hassle with the cumbersome burden of constantly counting the amount of calories, fats, and carbohydrates you consume. As you read through this book, you will discover how to effectively put each one of these seven key steps into action. The great part about using this approach to permanent weight loss is you won't have to deny yourself the foods you like or feel deprived like you would in most dieting programs.

People often panic when hunger pangs hit them, and they wreck their diets by binge eating on whatever foods they can get their hands on. Fortunately, my approach is not a diet, but a lifestyle change. No going under the surgeon's knife or taking diet pills. You will be able to eat and enjoy your favorite foods and deserts; I'll just teach you the best way to combine and eat them. You will learn how to avoid the common mistakes most people make when it comes to proper nutrition. This approach has been proven scientifically to be the most effective way to lose weight and keep it off permanently. It also helps to reverse and prevent many degenerative diseases that are directly linked to excessive weight. It's finally time to take control of your health, wealth and future. Educate and empower yourself with the knowledge that will change your life forever. Don't become another sad statistic, but make a difference instead and help someone else who is struggling to overcome.

WHY DIETING DOESN'T WORK

CHAPTER III

*S*adly, Americans spend an astronomical $40 to $50 billion annually on diet pills and weight loss products. Although some of these products do result in initial weight loss, it's not permanent, and the benefits come with a price. Common side effects from weight loss medications include nervousness, irritability, headaches, dry mouth, nausea, constipation, abdominal pain, diarrhea, sleep problems, intense dreams, and even heart problems.

What's really baffling is the medical community has clearly stated that obesity is a preventable cause of death resulting from unhealthy eating habits and a sedentary lifestyle. In other words, people can simply choose to modify their behavior and save their own lives and the lives of their precious loved ones. As I stated earlier, there are a myriad of different weight loss programs and products available on the market today, all touting to do basically the same thing: help us lose weight. There's the popular South Beach Diet, which according to research had the lowest ranking out of over 20 popular diets recently studied. Add to this the Atkins diet, Jenny Craig, L.A. Weight Loss Center and Weight Watchers, just to name a few.

There are myriads of weight loss meals like NutriSystem, Smart Choice, Smart ones, Healthy Choice, Lean Cuisine, Snackwells, and the endless supply of dietary health bars. Then there's the infinite number of so-called remarkable weight loss pills like Alli, which blocks the absorption of fat during digestion, but not without the unpleasant side effect like loose leaky stools. Some people using Alli reportedly had to actually wear diapers or carry around extra clothing for unexpected emergencies.

Everyone's hyped about the new wonder diet herb called Hoodia, which comes from the Kalahari Desert in Africa. The problem here is the people taking this diet drug do not live in the Kalahari, where there are some huge environmental differences that must be taken into consideration. For instance, the prevalence and unlimited availability of various types of highly refined and processed foods, coupled with a plethora of artificially sweetened sugary drinks, and the heavy usage of antibiotics and second hand antibiotic exposure through animal and dairy consumption. None of these conditions exist in the Kalahari, but they dominate the landscape of countries where the obesity epidemics are major problems.

Moving right along, there are diet drinks like Slim Fast, Ensure, diet colas, and diet teas, and while we're mentioning diet drinks, I want to point out something very interesting as it relates to their effectiveness: We all know that diet cola drinks have been around for quite some time now. In fact, Coca-Cola recently celebrated its' 25th anniversary in the lucrative diet cola business. But from the looks of things, it appears companies in the diet cola business are the only ones that have actually benefited over the past quarter century, with billions in profits. People have been faithfully buying and consuming these beverages for decades. Yet with all of the billions of dollars that have been spent by consumers thus far, none of these diet drink companies have been able to prevent people from gaining excessive amounts of weight, or even slightly stall the progressively growing global obesity pandemic.

From the way I look at it, if something is not a part of the solution, then it must be a part of the problem. This goes back to something I stated earlier, which has been confirmed by the experts: You're not going to find your weight loss miracle in a bottle of diet pills or in a can of diet cola. Now when all of these diet aids have failed to produce the desired results we had anticipated (that is losing weight, of course), we ultimately seek medical intervention and opt for procedures like liposuction, where doctors literally use a vacuuming device to suck fat from the body.

We also try options like gastric bypass surgery, which involves the removal of almost 95% of the stomach and 75% of the small intestine. There is also a surgical technique known as stomach stapling, which uses gastric staples to reduce the size of the stomach. Then there's mouth wiring, an oral weight control apparatus designed to block solid food from entering into the stomach.

Lastly, we have hypnosis and psychotherapy, age-old techniques designed to speak to the mind in an attempt to alter a person's behavior. On top of all this, it seems as though every month there are newly-discovered scientific findings as to why all these weight loss products haven't worked and people are continuing to gain weight.

Such scientific findings are usually followed by a newly manufactured magic diet pill concocted in some laboratory. Yes, almost every time you turn on your television set, there is a commercial touting the latest miracle weight loss product. But even with all of these products at our disposal, none of them seem to have put a dent in the growing obesity epidemic. As one researcher bluntly stated, if diets and diet products were really effective, there would be a lot more skinny people walking around. Amazingly, people are continuing to grow fatter and fatter with no end in sight. I often use the term "crippling" because obesity has now become the number one health threat to humans in this nation, and is spreading fast across the globe.

Consider the following current events recently reported in the media: For many decades doctors have administered medications via injections into the buttocks. However, recently scientists made a surprising discovery identifying a new problem directly related to obesity. At a conference hosted by the Radiological Society of North America, Dr. Victoria Chan, a researcher at the Adelaide and Meath Hospital in Dublin, published the results of her latest study. Her team of researchers discovered that obesity directly inhibited the effectiveness of injections by as much as 44% in men and an alarming 92% in women. She stated that the amount of fatty tissue overlying the muscles exceeded the length of the needles commonly used for injections.

Her work suggested that people who are overweight or obese are not receiving the maximum benefit of a drug, or receiving no benefit at all. If medication isn't properly absorbed into the blood stream, it remains in the fatty tissue causing local infection and irritation. Dr. Chan's report suggested that pharmaceutical companies would soon have to start manufacturing longer needles.

There is also the case of a mortuary crematorium in Sacramento, California that actually caught fire as a result of excessive amounts of fatty fluids that melted and leaked from an obese body during cremation. The fatty fluid became highly combustible and burst into flames. Firefighters were dispatched and quickly put the fire out.

Obesity is impacting the way autopsies are being performed in other countries like Australia. Pathologists are now requiring more heavy-duty autopsy facilities to handle obese corpses that are difficult to move and too heavy for standard-size trolleys and lifting hoists. These corpses pose logistical problems and notable occupational health and safety issues for mortuary staff. Professor Roger Byard, a pathologist at the University of Adelaide, stated that larger storage and dissection rooms and more robust equipment will be needed if Australia doesn't curb its obesity problem.

Professor Edward Janus reported the following results in the Medical Journal of Australia. He claimed that urgent action is required at the highest level to change unhealthy lifestyle habits by correcting diet, increasing physical activity and creating a more conducive environment to support these objectives. He concluded by stating that, in the future, Australia will need super-sized wheelchairs, ambulances, hospital beds, crematorium furnaces and, yes, even larger grave plots.

These new obesity challenges are not just affecting Australia; they're impacting other countries around the globe as well. Elsewhere, an obese teen aged girl has filed a lawsuit against an amusement park for kicking her off a roller coaster. She had not been allowed on the ride because she could not be safely strapped into her seat. Due to the enormous size of her upper torso, the overhead harnesses, which would normally prevent people from falling out of the ride, couldn't be forced into its locking mechanism. Consequently, the ride operator had to ask the young lady to leave the ride platform. I imagine she must have been very embarrassed being singled out in front of everyone on the ride that day.

A British woman wanting to start a new life with her husband in New Zealand was refused entry because according to Immigration officials she was too fat and would put a strain on the health care system. Initially they were both told they were too overweight and consequently banned from entering the country. However the husband, a former soldier with a Body Mass Index (BMI) of 42, lost enough weight to meet his visa requirements. Any BMI over 25 is considered unhealthy and overweight. Eventually the husband was granted permission to enter the country but his wife was unable to lose weight and was not granted entry. According to an endocrinologist for New Zealand's Fight the Obesity Epidemic, the country can't afford to import people who are going to significantly drain health resources. New Zealand's immigration website revealed that many other people had been banned for being obese.

New Zealand has implemented new strict guidelines for people trying to become citizens as it attempts to control the cost of treating obesity and related diseases. They now require that people be weighed upon receiving their visas in order to ensure they fall within the country's weight guidelines. Now you would think that, at some point, many of the roughly 70 million people in this country trying to lose weight would stop and say to themselves, if the last thousand or so weight loss products haven't worked thus far, why would I expect the next generation to be any more effective? The fact is, no amount of dieting, diet drugs, or medical intervention can replace, nor can they be an alternative to, healthy lifestyle changes. Fundamentally speaking, in order for people to experience successful, permanent, and tangible long-term weight loss results, they must modify their behavior mentally.

This profound statement is not just my own personal opinion, but the result of exhaustive research conducted by numerous government agencies, major universities, and large pharmaceutical conglomerates. According to government statistics and new scientific research, every weight loss program has failed miserably at producing permanent long-term tangible results. Recently, Dr. Traci Mann, associate professor of psychology at UCLA, stated that dieting does not lead to sustained weight loss or health benefits for the majority of people. Mann was the lead author of one of the most comprehensive and rigorous analyses of diets ever conducted, covering 31 long-term studies. Mann and her team of researchers recommended that Medicare should not fund weight loss programs as a treatment for obesity. They further stated that the benefits of dieting are too small and the potential harm is too large for dieting to be recommended as a safe, effective treatment for obesity. In the end, their study recommended the same advice that I have followed for almost 30 years:

Adopting healthier behaviors related to proper nutrition and routine exercises are the key factors to sustained weight loss. In fact, according to Professor Mann, studies consistently reveal that people who exercised more also shed the most pounds. You don't need a PhD to look around and see that people, regardless of their ethnicity, gender, age or economic status, are continuing to grow fatter by the burger.

Everywhere you look you can easily notice there are more overweight people than there are normal sized people. I'm sure you personally know many people who are currently dieting or have recently tried dieting, and who ultimately failed and simply gave up trying. Here is the frightening fact about yo-yo dieting: Evidence suggests that repeatedly losing and gaining weight is linked to cardiovascular disease, stroke, diabetes and altered immune function.

Here's another surprising discovery: One of the best predictors of weight gain is having previously lost weight on a diet. In fact, several studies have revealed that people who did not diet in many cases were better off than those who did diet. With all the latest advancements in medical science and technology over the past 70 years, there still appears to be no end in sight to the current obesity pandemic gripping this nation. I must reiterate; obesity and the enormous cost associated with treating obesity-related diseases are threatening the very financial stability of this country and nations around the globe as these nations adapt to the standard western diet of overly-processed foods and sugary drinks, which are nutrient-deficient and contain unhealthy fats and calories,

Recently, several popular marketers of weight-loss drugs were fined $25 million by the Food and Drug Administration for making false advertising claims regarding rapid weight loss, metabolism acceleration and misleading consumers. Fines were levied against such marketers as Xenadrine EFX, One A Day, Weight Smart, CortiSlim, CortiStress, and TrimSpa.

Federal Trade Commission (FTC) Chairman Deborah Platt Majoras stated that people are not going to find weight loss in a bottle of pills, and that these companies would have to stop making false claims. Surprisingly, some of these diet products didn't even contain many of the ingredients that were listed on the labels. In one case in particular, marketers of the popular diet pill Xenadrine had a study that showed people who took a placebo actually lost more weight than those taking their diet pill. The company not only lacked studies to support their claim, but actually had documented evidence that conclusively supported just the opposite.

The Bayer Corp., based in Morristown, NJ, agreed to pay $3.2 million in civil penalties to settle their claims and agreed to stop producing ads that say multi-vitamins can increase metabolism. These companies are required by the FTC to back up their claims with science, and if they can't do that they can't make the claims. To generate more in sales, many of these products are marketed through infomercials with endorsements from famous Hollywood celebrities like Kirstie Alley, Valerie Bertinelli, and Anna Nicole Smith, and sports figures like Dan Marino. The FTC does not consider testimonials from individuals as a substitute for science, and this is what the public needs to understand. While some of these products may produce short-term weight loss success stories, they fall far short of addressing the underlying fundamental reasons why people gain weight.

Additionally, the aspect of modifying one's behavior as it relates to proper nutrition is totally ignored by these companies, which is of paramount importance if you are going to try to both lose weight and keep it off permanently. In fact, if you take time to read the fine print on the package or listen carefully to the commercials, all of them suggest the need for proper nutrition and exercise in conjunction with the use of their products.

However, they fail to instruct us on how to accomplish this and instead push their individual products. What would happen if, God forbid, due to an unexpected financial hardship, a person could no longer afford these products? Without being properly educated about the importance of incorporating healthy lifestyle habits along with their nutritional regimen, people would simply regain their weight, ultimately wasting untold fortunes and putting their health at further risk. The benefit of learning behavior modification techniques is the fact that they are recession-proof and work regardless of whatever financial situation a person may find their self in. The major reasons why diets fail at successfully producing tangible and long-term results for the average person is that people are not being taught how to properly modify their behavior mentally, as it relates to proper nutrition and incorporating healthier lifestyle habits.

I tell people all the time, if you change your mind, eventually your body will follow. I'll repeat it again; no dieting, diet drugs or medical surgeries can replace, nor can they be an alternative to, healthy lifestyle habits. In order for people to have any successful, permanent and long-term results, they must modify their behavior first and foremost. In fact, one of the largest pharmaceutical companies in the world, and maker of the first FDA approved diet-pill, stated that you won't lose weight in your sleep or shed pounds while continuing to eat anything you want. That's the sobering message from diet drug maker Glaxo Smith Kline.

The company further stresses the need for nutrition and exercise to be incorporated in conjunction with any weight loss drug program. Although their new diet pill is poised to create $1.5 billion in annual sales for the company, they have undeniably concluded that taking their diet pill alone is not a magic bullet weight loss cure. The average person has been generally mislead and misguided about good nutrition. The word "exercise" these days is like the black plague, and water has been replaced with sugary soft drinks and sweetened juices. No weight loss plan can effectively produce successful long term tangible results without addressing the following three areas:

Good nutrition, exercise, and proper hydration.

These three key fundamental areas of optimum health must be addressed and incorporated simultaneously if you are going to have a successful weight loss career. Being properly educated about nutrition ensures that the foods you chose to consume are nutrient-rich and properly balanced for optimum assimilation and elimination.

Aerobic exercises and resistance training help build lean muscle mass and increase metabolic activity, which makes gaining weight more difficult and shedding pounds much easier. Exercising also helps deplete the body of excess glucose and other toxins as well as reserves of glucose stored in the liver and muscles. This process detoxifies the liver, enabling it to burn fat faster and helping to evenly distribute fat throughout the body. Another critical aspect of physical activity occurs when the liver and muscles empty stored levels of glucose into the blood during exercise to be used by the body for energy. Drinking plenty of water instead of soda and other sweetened beverages is crucial because water is free of sugar, carbs and calories, thus ensuring we aren't overloading our bodies with excessive amounts of glucose. Having less glucose circulating in the blood for shorter periods of time enables the body to produce less insulin, ultimately preventing unwanted fat storage. Remember, carrying excess weight increases your chances of developing certain degenerative diseases like diabetes, hypertension, heart disease and some forms of cancer.

I personally witnessed two friends of mine lose a combined total of 55 pounds by employing this simple but effective behavior modification approach of consuming less sugar and fewer sugary beverages. They replaced sugary beverages in their diet with more water and started exercising. In fact, one of them was able to reverse his previously diagnosed pre-diabetes condition. My friends were totally amazed at the results they achieved by simply removing excess sugar from their diets and adding moderate exercise.

Sadly, the effects of unwanted weight gain can lead to many other devastating complications. Oftentimes, people undermine themselves, especially women, thinking they can jump-start their weight loss plan by skipping meals, particularly breakfast. Not only is this approach to losing weight totally ineffective, it is un-healthy and causes you to binge-eat later on in the day, resulting in even more unwanted weight gain. Consider the fact that when you wake up in the morning you haven't had anything to eat for at least 5-8 hours. While you slept your body was busy repairing itself from the prior day's damages and then regenerating itself for the next day's challenges.

By the time you wake up and get started your body is eagerly ready for a wholesome healthy meal to kick off the day. In fact, your body needs nourishment at this time or else it will think it is being starved. When the body senses a state of starvation, primitive mechanisms kick in, activating the production of certain survival hormones. The most powerful of these hormones is called ghrelin, which triggers the desire to eat more and causes the body to conserve fat. No matter how much a person weighs, when their ghrelin level rises, their hunger increases. It also increases when you lose weight, causing a sense of panic and resulting in you grabbing for anything you can find to eat. This invariably makes dieting more difficult causing you to eat more and gain back the weight you initially lost.

On the other hand there is leptin, a powerful hunger-vanquishing hormone that suppresses ghrelin production. Leptin is manufactured from fat found in the foods you consume. It suppresses ghrelin by signaling the brain to increase production of the satisfaction hormone serotonin. When serotonin levels increase, a satisfaction sensation is induced, causing hunger to gradually dissipate. In other words, there is a converse relationship between ghrelin and leptin. When food reaches your stomach your ghrelin levels begin to fall and your leptin levels start rising. As it passes to your intestines, other satiety hormones assist with digestion by sending messages to your brain that you are getting full and you start feeling content. Additionally, as you eat your stomach stretches, sending more messages to your brain that you've had enough to eat. At this point you should push the plate away. The average person, however, ignores these signals and continues eating.

Ghrelin is mainly controlled by what and when you eat. For example, the best food sources to suppress ghrelin activity are carbohydrates and proteins. Carbohydrates' impact on ghrelin is more effective, while proteins have a longer lasting effect. On the other hand, fats have a limited effect on ghrelin levels. Additionally, both significant weight loss and lack of sleep can elevate ghrelin levels as well. In a study, scientists gave both normal and overweight individuals ghrelin, even though they had just ate and were not hungry. During the experiment, both groups immediately became hungry and started experiencing intense hunger pangs. The appetite of the normal weight group increased by 20%, while that of the overweight group increased by an astonishing 70%.

Unfortunately, overweight people have the hardest time regulating their hunger hormones. Studies conducted by researchers on both humans and animals revealed that when the hormone ghrelin was induced, appetite increased voraciously, in some cases by as much as 80%. The good news is, as you modify your eating habits, your ghrelin levels gradually begin to adjust. This is why behavior modification is more effective than dieting, because it gives the body time to adapt to the new changes.

Before using this approach, I had been on every diet you could imagine. With all of the diets, I initially lost weight, but it was short lived, and before I knew it, I was right back where I had started plus a few extra pounds heavier. It was like traveling on a never-ending diet roller coaster, with my weight progressively reaching new highs, with the lows being fewer and further between. It was a very depressing time for me, especially as I watched other friends and relatives go through the same process. I was beginning to think there was no hope and that I was destined to become this other person I never wanted to be. With the extra pounds, my mobility was diminished and I lacked bountiful energy, which left me feeling tired and sluggish most of the time.

At the end of the day, you need to ask yourself following questions:

Do I really want to take diet drugs and weight loss aids for the rest of my life?

Are they reasonably feasible and practically sound solutions to long-term permanent weight loss success?

Do I want my children to become dependent on diet drugs for the rest of their lives, as well?

Is it safe for them and what are the long-term health risk and cost consequences?

What's going to happen if I am no longer able to pay for these diet products?

Will my children and I regain the few pounds we've already lost, possibly endangering our health and wasting untold fortunes?

When it comes to being healthy and fit the answer is very straight-forward. The experts say that there are no short cuts and that behavior modification is the only thing that really works. If you just want to look thin, then maybe dieting is enough temporarily, at least on a short-term basis. But if you want to actually be healthy, then exercise has to be an important component of your lifestyle. Remember, according to all the available research, dieting and weight loss aids are not effective in producing long-term weight loss results.

With all that said, I hope you are beginning to see why, if you want a feasible, economical, and practical long-term approach to permanent weight loss, behavior modification techniques are absolutely crucial. This book is intended to teach you how to lose weight safely and effectively, with long-lasting permanent results. The greatest benefit about this approach is the fact that these techniques can be taught to other family members and friends as well, positively impacting their lives for generations. This book will teach you the behavior modification techniques that really work. Again, it's never too late, so why not get started today?

OBESITY & CHRONIC DISEASES

CHAPTER IV

Did you know?
- Obesity is the second leading preventable cause of death after smoking, killing 300,000 people annually.
- Being overweight or obese increases the risk of hypertension, heart disease, stroke, diabetes, cancer, and 30 other diseases.
- Almost 18% of boys and girls between the ages of 2-9 in the U.S. are overweight or obese.
- Approximately 127 million adults in the U.S. are Overweight; 60 million are obese and 9 million are severely obese.
- Obesity and related health problems drain an astronomical $117 billion annually from the U.S. economy.
- Americans spend between $40 and $50 billion annually on weight-loss products and related services.

*O*besity, as previously asserted, in an equal-opportunity epidemic that has become a problem on a global scale and poses one of the greatest threats to human health and well-being in the 21st century. Obesity has now been changed from a minor to a major risk factor for coronary heart disease by the American Heart Association. The other major risk factors are smoking, high blood pressure, high cholesterol, and a sedentary lifestyle. You may not have had the time to read the latest troubling headlines about obesity: Researchers are predicting that if people keep increasing in size and nothing is done, obesity will not only be the norm by the year 2015, it will be the leading preventable cause of death in the United States and around the world.

By then, according to experts, it's expected that 75% of the adults living in the U.S. will be overweight, and almost half will be obese. This means that every 3 out of 4 adults will be at risk for developing one or more of 30 medical conditions known to be caused by obesity. It's unfathomable even trying putting a price tag on dealing with such an enormous problem. According to Dr.

William Dietz of the Centers for Disease Control and Prevention in Atlanta, further complicating matters is the fact that many people are unlikely to admit the severity of their weight problems for fear of being seen in a negative light.

The medical definition of obesity is a condition in which the natural energy reserves, stored in the fatty tissue of humans and other mammals, are increased to a point that is associated with certain health conditions or increased mortality. Obesity is both an individual clinical condition and is increasingly viewed as a serious public health problem. Excessive body weight has been shown to predispose us to various diseases, particularly cardiovascular diseases, diabetes mellitus Type 2, sleep apnea, and osteoarthritis. Through change in diet and increased physically activity, these diseases are preventable.

Even modest weight loss can bring significant improvements in health and a reduction in the level of risk. It appears as though the culprit is the Standard American Diet (SAD). You can literally follow SAD's trail, as wherever it goes, obesity and related diseases are sure to follow. As more and more cultures around the globe start replacing their traditional healthy diets with SAD, they are starting to see dramatic increases in the rates of obesity and obesity-related diseases such as diabetes, hypertension, and heart disease.

Today, the standard medical professional method for determining if someone is overweight is known as the Body Mass Index (BMI). BMI is the ratio between height and weight in kilograms per meter squared. Obesity is defined as having a BMI of 30 or more. The normal BMI range is between 8.5 and 24.9, while the overweight range is 25 to 29.9, and severe obesity is 40 or more. If your BMI is 25 or higher, you could be at risk for high blood pressure, high cholesterol, heart disease, stroke, diabetes, arthritis, menstrual disturbances, lower-back pain, skin problems, and psychological disorders.

In real estate, the best deals are determined by the location of the property being bought or sold. "Location, location, location!" is the term commonly used. The same idea applies to fat, as the location of fat storage can either work to your advantage or to your detriment. Depending on where the fat is located, it can help protect against diabetes, heart disease and hypertension, or help cause these same diseases.

Body fat comes in two different varieties: subcutaneous fat, a noticeable layer of fat that lies just below the skin, and visceral fat, which is invisibly buried beneath the muscle. Subcutaneous fat comprises 80% of bodily fat cells and are stored in the squishy areas just beneath the skin of your buttocks, thighs, upper arms, chest and stomach. This type of fat isn't harmful, although the same cannot be said for visceral fat, which comprises the remaining 20% of fat cells in the body and poses the greatest health risk. Visceral fat surrounds the major organs and muscles. Too much of it stored in these areas can be unhealthy; it can clog your arteries and drain into your liver, impairing this vital organ.

Research shows that people who consume large amounts of saturated fat and perform little or no exercise are likely to have high stores of visceral fat. The smaller your waistline, the more likely it is that you are not carrying a large buildup of visceral fat. In fact, the only effective way to view this fat is through Magnetic Resonance Imaging (MRI), which uses magnetic waves to take pictures of the inside of the abdomen.

Most women store fat in their hips, buttocks, and thighs, while most men store fat around their mid-section. While a standard BMI reading will not determine how much visceral fat you may be carrying around, many studies have found that waist circumference is a more valuable tool at determining how much unhealthy visceral fat a person has. Women with a waist circumference greater than 88 cm are more than likely carrying around dangerous amounts of visceral fat.

Some of the fat that sticks around our internal organs secretes a form of estrogen in both men and women. In overweight females who haven't yet experienced menopause, the extra estrogen may reduce the risk of osteoporosis. However, it may also increase the risk of breast cancer. Overweight males should be cautious too, because the excess estrogen can give them larger breasts and make them impotent. Scientists theorize that internal fat surrounding the organs disrupts the body's ability to communicate effectively. The fat might be sending the body mistaken chemical signals to store fat inside organs like the liver and pancreas. Ultimately, this could lead to insulin resistance, heart disease, and Type 2 diabetes.

It has been known for some time that active fat people can be healthier than inactive skinny people. People, who are sedentary and unfit, even if they are not overweight, are at a much higher risk for disease and death than active obese people, according to obesity experts. The good news is visceral fat is easier to burn off than subcutaneous fat through exercise and a healthy diet: two key components of the behavior modification techniques taught in this book. Just exercising moderately most days of the week can help prevent the build-up of visceral fat. Bouts of vigorous exercise, such as walking, swimming and playing tennis, can markedly reduce the amount of visceral fat you already have.

Currently, an alarming 80% of African American women aged 40 or over are overweight and 50% are obese. Sixteen percent of U.S. children and adolescents are overweight, and 34% are at risk of becoming overweight, according to federal government figures. In a recent Associated Press news poll, when asked which health risk posed the greatest danger to Americans today, terrorism was not at the top of the list. Instead an overwhelming majority of the respondents stated un-healthy eating habits posed the greatest risk. Before I proceed further, I want to briefly explain a few things about fat and how it works in the body. This will help you understand a little more clearly the relationship between excessive weight and the development of chronic degenerative diseases that are directly related to obesity.

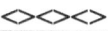

Fat Basics

Most people have an unhealthy misconception about fat and are generally misguided to believe that all fat is bad for you. Some have even tried dangerously removing fats totally from their diets, thinking this would make them much healthier and leaner. We have been led to believe for decades that all fats are the same, with some people actually fearing fat like a deadly plague. Fat has been blamed for causing everything from obesity to cancer to diabetes to heart disease. The truth is, not all fat is bad for you and without some good fats like essential fatty acids in our diets your bodies wouldn't function at all.

Fat is actively involved in every bodily function you can imagine: brain function, hormone production, oxygen and nutrient transport into cells, immune system function, nervous system activity, glandular function, hemoglobin production, intra-cellular communication, protecting cells against foreign bodies, proper digestion, assimilation of nutrients, and stopping allergens. More important than vitamins, minerals, and even proteins, without essential fatty acids, there is no life. Fats are responsible for helping us hear, see, move our muscles, and breathe; they aid in blood vessel constriction, heart regulation, and many more bodily functions. In the absence of fat, you wouldn't be able to scan the pages of this book or lift weights while exercising. Believe it or not, I know this may sound a bit crazy, but fat is also responsible for helping to maintain proper body weight.

What you may not realize is that fat is nothing more than stored energy. After you have eaten a meal, the fat from your food is transformed into fatty acids by the trillions of friendly bacteria living in your colon. They also transform protein into amino acids, carbohydrates into glucose, and are responsible for the proper storage of these essential nutrients in the body. Once the fatty acids are manufactured they're either used immediately or the body stores them in reserve to be used another day. This is where one of the problems with excessive weight begins; because most people don't exercise regularly, another day never actually materializes. In essence, in the absence of exercise, a person is simply storing fat on top of fat with each and every additional meal. When fat is not in use by the body, it is stored in fat cells. Fat cells are like tiny balloons that have the capacity to increase almost 100 times in weight and volume. When fat cells are stretched to their limit, signals are sent out to the surrounding tissue to produce new fat cells. It is easy to understand how a person can easily become overweight if he or she is not using up stored fat reserves.

A certain group of fats known as essential fatty acids are contained mostly in polyunsaturated oils and are vitally important to maintaining optimum health. Not only are these essential fats good for you, they have been proven scientifically to help reverse heart disease, hypertension, diabetes, and obesity. In fact, several studies have indicated that olive oil, in addition to being good for your heart can actually help you lose weight. Recent research is now revealing that fat in general is not the problem, but is the type of fat that is the real culprit. The unhealthy fats, known as omega-6 fatty acids are responsible for many painful inflammatory conditions such as asthma, eczema, psoriasis, rheumatoid arthritis, ulcerative colitis, Crohn's disease, lupus, multiple sclerosis, and many more. Omega-6 fatty acids produce inflammatory chemicals like leukotrienes, prostaglandin, and thromboxanes that are made from food fat, specifically, meat, dairy products, cooking oils, corn oil, margarine, salad oils, safflower oils, and sunflower oil.

Deadly man-made hydrogenated fats belong in a class all by themselves, as they contribute to a whole host of deadly diseases and are now being banned from use in our foods. On the other hand, fats like Omega-3 fatty acids are essential for good health and produce anti-inflammatory chemicals like docosahexaenioc acid (DHA) and eicosapentaenoic acid (EPA). Both of these chemicals counteract and neutralize inflammatory disease-causing prostaglandin and leukotrienes. EPA has been scientifically proven to be crucial in preventing heart disease, and DHA is important for optimum brain function.

Although we need both Omega-3 and 6 fatty acids, their unbalanced ratio causes most of our health problems. For example, a healthy normal ratio of Omega-3 to Omega-6 fatty acids should be a balance of 7 Omega-3 to 3 Omega-6 fatty acids. However, with the SAD consisting of highly-refined and overly-processed foods, this balance is dangerously altered to an unhealthy ratio of 21 Omega-6 to only 2 Omega-3 fatty acids. This unhealthy imbalance allows the inflammatory Omega-6 fatty acids to go unchecked. While inflammatory responses are naturally needed in our bodies, too much of this response becomes unhealthy. It's sort of like leaving your bath water on after the tub is full; eventually water will spill over and cause all kinds of damage to your home. Without the proper counter-balancing of anti-inflammatory Omega-3 fatty acids in their proper ratio, the inflammatory chemicals wreak all kinds of havoc in our bodies.

I mentioned earlier that fat cells have an incredible ability to stretch in size by almost 100% in volume. It was once thought that everyone was born with a predetermined number of fat cells, however new research has revealed just the opposite. We actually produce new fat cells throughout our entire lifetime. Many think they can permanently remove fat through surgery but this belief is misguided. There are obese people who have lost weight by having gastric bypass surgery and liposuction, only to end up gaining it back again, because they failed to change their eating habits, which, by the way, takes us right back to behavior modification techniques, as without this component one can never permanently lose weight.

To begin with, these behavior modification techniques ensure that your fat cells never end up reaching their stretching capacity. If fat cells don't become engorged, the body doesn't produce new fat cells, enabling you to permanently maintain your weight naturally. While a normal-sized person can have roughly 40 billion fat cells, an obese person can have more than twice as many. Many people think that fat cells just lazily hang around and do nothing, but that is not the case. Fat is actually a great big gland, producing hormones and other chemical substances that are essential to many bodily functions.

Researchers have discovered more than 100 biochemical substances that fat produces called adipokines. Most of these adipokines cause inflammation in tissues and blood vessels, and if left unchecked increase the risk of both heart attack and stroke. These substances can make our bodies resistant to insulin raising the risk of developing diabetes mellitus Type 2. They can also elevate blood pressure and raise the risk of developing blood clots.

A hormone called adiponectin helps the body respond positively to insulin and minimizes fat's ability to clog arteries. Unfortunately, the more weight you gain the less of this hormone your body produces. With all that you have just read about fat it is clearly to your advantage to manage your weight and avoid many of the complications associated with obesity. It is also just as imperative to incorporate sources of healthy fats into your diet that are beneficial in reducing inflammation.

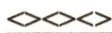

Intestinal Dysbiosis:
Most of us cringe when we hear the word bacteria and immediately imagine deadly microscopic germs. We go to great lengths to make sure we exclusively purchase antibacterial cleansers, body washes, soaps, lotions and a myriad of other products that are designed to totally wipe out all bacteria. We want everything in our environment to be perfectly clean, safe and absolutely free of any

type of bad germs. When we come down with certain ailments, antibiotics are prescribed to help destroy the bacteria responsible for causing our illnesses. We are constantly bombarded by the scientific community with pejorative reports about dangerous and deadly bacterial outbreaks.

Rarely do we ever hear any positive news about bacteria and how they are actually beneficial to our health and can sometimes be more potent than antibiotics at treating some diseases. What we fail to understand is that without these beneficial strains of bacteria, there is no such thing as a perfect environment, good health, or the existence of life as we know it. This general misconception has to do with the fact that the average person has been misinformed about the positive role certain bacteria play in helping to keep us alive and healthy. There are various types of friendly (healthy) and unfriendly (unhealthy) bacteria that thrive within our bodies and in our environment. They are inescapable and have been around for billions of years.

Human breast milk contains lactose sugar that protects infants by helping them colonize healthy levels of friendly bacteria like Bifidobacteria and Lactobacilli. These bacteria restrict colonization of disease-causing organisms. There are more than 400 different strains of several hundred trillion friendly bacteria living in our colon area at any given time. In fact, there are more bacteria living in our bodies than there are cells that make up who we are. As you probably already know, America is a vitamin and supplement-taking nation. We use supplements for just about everything you can imagine. However, no amount of vitamins, no matter how expensive or potent they may be, can be fully assimilated and benefit your body unless they are first broken down by our friendly intestinal bacteria. These beneficial bacteria support the lining of the GI tract, which is essential for nutrient absorption and for maintaining optimal pH levels in the colon by making organic acids.

I'm sorry to burst your bubble, but you are just throwing away your money without the proper level of these beneficial bacteria living in your colon. In order for you to receive the full maximum benefit of supplements, you must first correct the balance of intestinal flora (friendly bacteria). These bacteria are responsible for manufacturing and aiding in the digestion of all vitamins, especially B-vitamins, including B12 and folic acid. These bacteria assist in the production and preservation of essential fatty acids, breaking down lactose (milk sugars) and protein, cleansing the intestinal tract, purifying the colon, and maintaining regular bowel movements. They protect us from environmental toxins, rebuild hormones, help maintain healthy cholesterol levels, manage and destroy harmful bacteria, molds, viruses and parasites, prevent infection, and create lactic acid. In fact, the folate in the food you eat must first be converted into folic acid by friendly bacteria before it can be used by the body.

Imagine for a moment that your body is a gigantic food distribution warehouse serving a large metropolis. You are responsible for delivering food products to various schools, hospitals, restaurants, and other establishments in the area you serve. Every day, millions of tons of products are brought into your warehouse from all over the country for redistribution. As these items are unloaded and inventoried, armies of warehouse workers process orders for various customers. However, before these products can be shipped out, they must be broken down first and then repackaged into smaller-sized packages to meet the specific needs of each individual client. This momentous task is accomplished by the millions of warehouses workers who feverishly work 24 hours a day making sure customers get the right products.

This is exactly what healthy bacteria do in your body. As food(like chicken, ribs, steaks, fruits, and vegetables) comes in, this vast army of bacteria breaks down the food into the proper chemical compounds, and then repackages it for distribution throughout the body. Ninety percent of these friendly bacteria line your intestinal walls, where they help to keep your immune system vibrant and in optimum working condition. They help aid with the digestion, assimilation, and elimination of the various foods we consume daily.

For centuries, scientists have known about the positive role healthy bacteria play in treating diseases, and have even used them to treat various ailments. The bacteria L. Gasseri, for example, is more beneficial at protecting us from the common H. Pylori bacteria, known to cause stomach ulcers, than most over-the-counter and prescription medications. Recently, immunologists at the University of Naples Federico II in Italy experimented using viruses that are harmless to humans to kill a drug-resistant superbug bacteria. This superbug causes the deadly form of Staphylococcus Aureus (the cause of staph infections), commonly found in U.S. hospitals. The microbe, dubbed MRSA, evolved over time and became resistant to commonly used antibiotics. However, by introducing friendly bacteria that prey on the Staphylococcus Aureus, scientists were able to completely neutralize the virus, which was 97% effective at destroying the MRSA superbug.

Ideally, 85% of the roughly four pounds of resident bacteria in the colon should be beneficial strains, with the remaining 15% being hostile bacteria. The friendly bacteria are mostly aerobic, which means they flourish in an oxygen-rich environment. The hostile bacteria are anaerobic, meaning they thrive and flourish in absence of oxygen. When useful strains of bacteria are reduced below 85%, an imbalance (dysbiosis) occurs. One of the main causes of this imbalance is antibiotics, or exposure to second-hand antibiotics, such as those found in non-organic meat, poultry, fish, eggs, and dairy products. This is why it is so important to consume organic foods, as they are free of unnecessary antibiotics and pesticides. Other causes are radiation, chlorinated water, steroids, unhealthy diet, refined sugar, oral contraceptives, unmanaged stress, diarrhea and cold medicines.

An imbalance can greatly inhibit digestion, causing poor elimination and the storage of several pounds of putrefying toxic waste. Hostile bacteria will cause all kinds of havoc as they travel via the blood throughout the entire body, damaging tissues, arteries and cells. For example, sometimes the bacteria Candida albicans, commonly known for its role in causing yeast infections, will travel outside the colon area. As they travel throughout the body they release powerful poisons called cytotoxins. Common symptoms of cytotoxin poisoning are headaches, allergies, constipation, fatigue, gas, muscle aches, insomnia, vaginal discharge, itching, PMS, asthma, weight problems, psoriasis, eczema, acne, and sinus problems.

You have probably never made the direct connection between a healthy intestinal bacterial balance and excess weight, but all the evidence is there. In fact, it has been scientifically proven than non-breast fed infants are more likely to be obese when they become teens than breast-fed infants. One reason for this phenomenon is the fact that the intestinal bacteria of non-breast fed teens has never been fully developed and normally remains unbalanced for most of their lives. People definitely have the option to choose to practice healthier habits promoting good health. Making the right choices can greatly improve the chances of preventing over 30 obesity-related diseases. I want to briefly list some of the common diseases associated with obesity here and explain a few of them in more detail below:

An overweight person can develop depression, diabetes, hypertension, various forms of cancer, cardiovascular disease, impaired respiratory function, liver disease, morbid obesity, pancreatitis, infertility, rheumatoid arthritis, end stage renal disease, osteoarthritis, birth defects, gout, gallbladder disease, carpal tunnel syndrome, low back pain, daytime sleepiness, deep vain thrombosis, heat disorders, impaired immune response, obstetric and gynecologic complications, pain, sleep apnea, stroke, heel spurs, premature aging and surgical complications, abdominal hernias, gastroesophagal reflux and lower-extremity edema.

Obesity and Diabetes

Nearly 20 million Americans have diabetes; approximately 10 million of these individuals are totally unaware that they suffer from the disease. There are two main types of diabetes: Type I diabetes which reportedly accounts for roughly 7% of all diagnosed cases. Most often it appears in childhood or adolescence and causes high blood sugar when your body can't make enough insulin. The remaining 93% of the diagnosed cases is Type 2 diabetes. Years ago, Type 2 diabetes was usually diagnosed in people forty or older, however, today it is showing up in people of all ages including infants, children, and adolescents. Both obesity and a sedentary lifestyle have been directly linked to Type 2 diabetes. People with Type 2 diabetes make insulin, but their bodies don't properly utilize it.

Initially, your body produces excessive amounts of insulin to keep blood sugar levels normal. However, over time the pancreas becomes overworked and can't produce enough insulin to keep blood sugars in a normal range. Perpetually elevated blood sugar levels ultimately lead to diabetes. Over an extended period of time, high blood sugar levels and diabetes can cause heart disease, stroke, blindness, kidney failure, leg and foot amputations, and pregnancy complications. Look at the snowball effect and insidiousness of obesity as it slowly robs a person of their health.

Diabetes is nothing to play with, as over 200,000 people die each year from diabetes-related complications. Excessive body weight and body fat are directly tied to the development of Type 2 diabetes. Overweight people are at a much greater risk of developing Type 2 diabetes than normal weight individuals. In fact almost 90% of people suffering from Type 2 diabetes are overweight. In the 1990s, the number of diabetes cases among American adults increased by one third and it is expected to continue climbing. It appears as though this rapid in-crease in diabetes is due to the growing prevalence of obesity and extra weight in the United States population, and is spreading fast around the globe. It has been medically proven that Type 2 diabetes is totally preventable and in many cases reversible. Research studies have found that lifestyle changes and small amounts of weight loss can prevent or delay the development of Type 2 diabetes among high-risk adults.

These lifestyle changes are the behavior modification techniques taught in this book. Behavior modification, including nutrition and moderately-intensive physical activities like brisk walking, jogging, and swimming, can produce small amounts of weight loss. In most cases, diabetes can be reversed or greatly marginalized with the loss of just 10% of total body weight. Managing your weight is the best thing you can do to prevent the development of diabetes. Weight management and exercise can positively impact your blood sugar levels and overall health. Using behavior modification tools like proper nutrition, hydration, routine exercise, managing stress, and incorporating lifestyle changes can significantly lower the cost associated with diabetic medications. Small amounts of weight reduction can decrease the amount of medication required to keep your blood sugar in the healthy range.

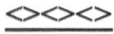

Obesity and Hypertension

Obesity is reported to be directly attributed to over 75% of high blood pressure or hypertension cases in this United States. Weight or BMI in association with age is the strongest indicator of hypertension in humans. Obese adult Americans between the ages of 23 to 46 are five to six times more likely to develop hypertension compared to non-obese adults of the same age. A blood pressure level of 140 (systolic) over 90 (diastolic) or more is considered serious enough to require being seen by your physician. Research suggests elevated BMI levels can increase the risk of ischemic stroke, independent of other risk factors including age and systolic blood pressure. Men who carry excess abdominal weight appear to be at greater risk of suffering from a stroke, and women who are overweight or who become obese are at a higher risk of suffering from an ischemic stroke as well.

Worldwide, approximately 1 billion people suffer from hypertension, and another half billion will be impacted by this silent killer by the year 2025. Hypertension is not just a problem in the ever-fattening Western world; it is even being felt in parts of Africa. This translates into more than two million deaths each year from heart disease alone. High blood pressure is the leading cause of strokes. Hypertension also plays a role in blindness and even dementia, but patients seldom notice these symptoms until organs have already been damaged.

Improving diet and exercising can help tremendously in managing and reversing this disease. In many African American churches, hypertension has become a Sunday service sermon topic. High blood pressure affects nearly one in three adults in this country, or roughly 72 million people. Unfortunately, anyone can get high blood pressure, even young children. I personally know of several adolescents and children as young as 5 years of age who currently take high blood pressure medication.

Obesity and Cancer

Being overweight and having an elevated BMI can put you at risk of developing various types of cancers that are directly linked to obesity. They include but are not limited to esophageal, colorectal, endometrial, prostate, breast, and renal cell cancers. Being overweight dramatically raises the risk of developing several forms of cancer in both men and women. Researchers recently studied women who gained weight as adults, and found that they face a higher lifetime risk of all types of breast cancer. According to their research and the large body of evidence available, weight and breast cancer appear to be closely linked. Researchers studied more than 44,000 women and found that the more weight a woman gained, the greater was her risk for breast cancer in all categories such as types, stages, and grades. They compared women who gained 20 pounds or less during adulthood to women who gained more than 20 pounds during adulthood. The researchers found that women who gained more than 60 pounds were twice as likely to have breast tumors and an increase in lobular type cancers.

Women who gained more than 60 pounds tripled the chance of their cancer spreading. Breast cancer risk is also linked to increased levels of the hormone estrogen, which is produced by fat tissue. Pre-menopausal women diagnosed with breast cancer who are overweight appear to have a shorter life span than women with a lower BMI. The undeniable link between excess weight and breast cancer further stresses the importance of maintaining a healthy body weight throughout adulthood. It is estimated that more than 200,000 people are diagnosed with breast cancer and roughly 40,000 die annually from this deadly obesity related disease annually here in the United States. Also, this is not just a disease that impacts females; globally more than 1.2 million men and women develop breast cancer every year. This topic is too large for me to cover in greater depth however there are numerous publications and books available regarding the extensive relationship between obesity and cancer.

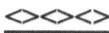

Obesity Related Depression
There is no doubt that people who are overweight are also more likely to be depressed because of their condition. Every overweight person I have ever known, including children, family and friends, have all dealt with bouts of depression as a result of being overweight. Obesity-related depression seems to be more prevalent among adolescents as they try to fit in with the social cliques

amongst their peer groups. In social settings, obese people tend to be singled out more for jokes and harassment. This can be devastating for a young, vulnerable, insecure teen. This is also the time when youngsters become sexually attracted to one another with most being concerned about their appearance. Many obese people suffer from rejection during this time of their lives, and they are more likely to deal with bouts of obesity-related depression during this time as well.

This is a very sensitive time that can lead to an increase in suicide attempts. People are designed to be sociable by nature and most desire to be accepted within certain peers groups. Of all the diseases associated with obesity, depression, in my opinion, is probably the worst one. I say this only because unlike heart disease, diabetes and hypertension, which are all internal and physically invisible to the naked eye, obesity is physically visible and as inescapable as your own shadow. Twenty-four hours a day, 7 days a week, 365 days a year, obese people are constantly reminded about their weight. In almost every aspect of their lives, from buying clothes to getting a job, they have to make adjustments for their excessive weight. It is this constant visual and physical awareness that I believe can cause the most damage and further exacerbate the other life-threatening conditions.

Depression causes certain chemical reactions in the body that release harmful hormones. These hormones, combined with other obesity-related inflammatory conditions, can rapidly deteriorate a person's health. Most people don't take being embarrassed very well, increasing the likelihood of them having to deal with obesity-related depression. Obesity also causes an imbalance in chemicals that regulate how a person feels. Scientifically, there is a definite connection between how much a person weighs and how that person feels.

Obese people often feel isolated and have a harder time making it up the corporate ladder, despite how qualified they may be. Overall, obesity just isn't attractive to most people, as talk show host Tyra Banks proved by going under cover disguised as an obese 300 pound woman. She had camera crews follow her around as they secretly documented how people interacted with an obese person. Even though she was not obese in real life, the experience brought her to tears as she experienced first-hand the type of public rejection, harassment, and humiliation obese people have to endure. It's hard enough for a person of normal weight to deal with rejection; now imagine being 200 pounds or more overweight.

It has been well-documented that people who lose weight suffer from fewer bouts of obesity-related depression. Since obese children are teased more often, this social stigmatization can cause obesity-related depression due to feelings of guilt, shame and embarrassment. Parents should closely monitor their children's weight and teach them how to modify their behavior around food and health in general so that they can avoid these unnecessary experiences.

Obesity and Heart Disease

The link between heart disease and obesity has been well established for decades. Physicians constantly advise their overweight heart patients to lose weight, watch what they eat, and exercise moderately. Heart disease is mostly preventable or can be greatly reduced. It is the result of poor nutritional habits and a sedentary lifestyle. Obesity raises LDL ("bad") cholesterol and triglyceride levels, and decreases HDL ("good") cholesterol. This leads to heart disease, and its effects can begin in childhood. Overweight and obese children are at an even greater risk of developing coronary heart disease as they grow older. Weight loss improves blood lipid levels by lowering triglycerides and LDL cholesterol and increasing HDL cholesterol.

Obesity is a major risk factor for heart disease because it harms both the heart and blood vessel system, which can lead to a heart attack. Some reasons for this higher risk are known, but others are not. This is frightening when you consider that 1 out of every 3 Americans is obese. Excess weight is associated with several forms of heart disease and can be linked to some heredity factors as well. Diets high in saturated fats mostly from animal and dairy products and reduced physical activities are most likely the causes. Although most of the complications related to obesity and heart disease rise as BMI increases, they also relate to body fat dispersal. Extensive research indicates that coronary atherosclerosis is not only related to, but can be independently predicted by, obesity. This relationship appears to exist for both men and women, even if there is no increase in BMI.

As obesity adversely impacts the function of the left ventricular chamber of the heart, it increases cardiac output and diastolic dysfunction. These changes in the left ventricle are related to sudden death in obese patients. As body weight increases, the heart undergoes tremendous stress because it constantly has to beat harder to pump more blood. Over time, obesity can cause obstructive sleep apnea and/or right ventricular hypoventilation syndrome. As such conditions progress, they can eventually lead to heart failure and death. When obesity adversely impacts both the right and left ventricle, the heart failure that develops is called biventricular. This relationship may be cause-and-effect, in that when body weight increases, so does the increase risk for coronary heart diseases.

On the other hand, when weight decreases so does the associated risk. The best way to avoid heart disease is to balance the ratio of heart-healthy essential fatty acids, while avoiding unhealthy fats. It is also important to eat whole grain foods, minimize sugar intake and exercise moderately. These are just a few steps you can implement today to start improving the condition of your heart. Consult with your family physician who will be better able to help you with any existing heart problems.

THE FAT GENE THEORY

CHAPTER V

*T*here are a myriad of opinions and theories circulating around today as to why it is impossible for some people to lose weight, or why some tend to have a harder time than others and eventually give up trying. Why is it, for example, some people who say they eat very little food mysteriously and effortlessly gain massive amounts of weight? Such individuals say they're afraid to even look at food for fear that by doing so it will trigger the onset of this strange weight gaining phenomenon.

Researchers have gone so far as to say that unwanted weight gain may be caused by a genetic disorder certain people are born with. Others in the scientific community speculate it may be the result of some type of mental disorder or a mysterious hormone that causes a person to spontaneously gain weight. To further complicate matters, there is the recently discovered "fat gene" equation to throw into the mix, which, in my honest opinion, simply makes losing weight a much more difficult matter. Some of these impossible-to-lose-weight myths are further broken down by genetics, postulating that a person's propensity to become obese is connected to a family history of obesity.

Even though science is just beginning to uncover various possibilities, the newly-discovered hormones and genes making news headlines today were with us some 70 years ago when the word obesity was virtually unheard of. You may wonder why I don't buy into these theories, and it may sound like I am a bit insensitive. But before you pass judgment and stop reading this book, consider the following well-documented fact:

In third world countries around the globe, where food is not available in abundance, and overly-processed fast food and snacks are not sold, obesity and obesity-related diseases and are virtually non-existent. In fact, there are no overweight or obesity epidemics affecting 1 out every 3 people, as is the case in developed western countries. There are no weight loss centers or clinics like Jenny

Craig, L.A. Weight Loss, or Curves. These impoverished nations are not experiencing an obesity epidemic of any kind whatsoever.

Again, the overabundance and excessive consumption of highly-processed foods, refined sugar and artificial sweeteners are major contributing factors to this problem. In countries where there is an abundance of these types of foods, obesity and obesity related diseases are increasing to unprecedented historical levels. When processed and fast foods are unavailable, there appear to be two positive benefits: First, the population is leaner and healthier, and secondly, there are less chronic diseases associated with obesity like diabetes, hypertension, heart disease, and about 30 other obesity related diseases. Now you might disagree with me, but believe it or not, today more people around the globe die each year from having too much food than all those who die from having too little. In fact, the number of deaths associated with obesity dramatically trumps the combined total of all deaths of malnourished people around the globe. I'm in no way advocating starvation or malnutrition I'm just using this contrast to make a point.

A recent study released by the International Society for the Study of Obesity stated that both obesity and diabetes, which are directly associated with excessive weight gain, affects some 300 million people worldwide, and this twin epidemic will be responsible for shortening life expectancy around the world. It appears as though the more body weight you carry around, the shorter time you'll likely have to carry it. These figures do not include the millions of other people currently living in developed countries who eventually will be impacted by one or more of the 30 other obesity-related diseases.

Today, roughly 70% of this country's population is overweight and 35% are clinically obese. Authorities now agree that the average American diet no longer provides the needed nutrition for a foundation of good health. In this country of good and plenty, it appears as though plenty may not be all that good. In fact, as the dietary habits of western countries start to reach developing countries, obesity and obesity-related diseases are starting to rise exponentially. Recent research has revealed that the astronomical cost of treating obesity and obesity-related diseases may actually threaten the financial stability of many developing countries. The only difference between developed and non-developed nations is the over-abundance and availability of food, coupled with a sedentary lifestyle. Also, in developed countries, people can eat as much as they want when-ever they feel like it. In other words, overexposure to anything in any environment can eventually become dangerous and hazardous to one's health.

For example, we all need water to survive however drinking too much water can be fatal. Fire is necessary for warmth and cooking, however being exposed to fire for an extended period of time will cause severe harm. The same applies to food. While we need it to nourish our bodies, over consumption can become hazardous to one's health, especially excess consumption of processed foods. In one experiment, scientists took normal-weight people along with obese people and separated them into two groups. No one in either of the groups was tested for various hormones. Each group had excessive amounts of food made available to them over a period of several days. To the surprise of the scientists, both groups consumed far more food and calories than they would have under normal conditions. The researchers concluded that by being exposed to more food than normal, each group unconsciously overate. It doesn't matter what type of genes a person has: less calories and fat, (particularly unhealthy fats and calories) along with routine exercise, equals less weight gain and obesity.

Although the so called "fat gene" was just recently discovered by scientists, it is still unclear how this gene works in the human body, and whether or not it can overtake the free-will of individuals, forcing them to compulsively over eat. Still there are other factors to consider: for instance, does this gene interact differently with certain types of foods? If so, how can it distinguish which foods to interact with? Also, does the fat gene take into account the amount of fats and carbohydrates a person consumes with each meal? I guess the most intriguing question one would have to ask is, where was this gene 40 years ago when the rate of obesity in developed countries, particularly the United States and the U.K., stood at only 12%?

Over the past 30 years, we have gone through major weight loss fads like the fat-free and low-fat 1980sand early 90s. When that didn't work, we targeted refined sugar and started the sugar-free war for the next decade. Around this time, refined sugar was replaced with artificial sweeteners, as it was believed that these sweeteners were the magic answer to the nation's weight problem. At the turn of the millennium, experts targeted carbohydrates as the culprit, and the low-carb craze went into full swing. What's amazing is that with all the weight loss fads previously mentioned, developed societies have continued to gain weight in epidemic proportions. The obesity problem has recently gotten the attention of the Federal Government, which has decided to step in and try to stem this seemingly unstoppable health crisis.

People were endangering their lives trying these weight loss fads by totally eliminating all carbohydrates and fats, which are imperative to optimum overall health. When you consider the non-existence of obesity and weight related problems in poor developing countries where food is not in abundance, and where the population as a whole is more active, you will see why I'm not an advocate of the newly discovered "fat gene" theory as being the culprit behind the obesity epidemic.

But don't just take my word for it we can simply compare the facts. As I stated earlier, weight loss companies are not clamoring to open franchises in underdeveloped third world countries, because they wouldn't have any clients. Companies are in business to make money and to do that they need customers. From the people starving to death in Communist North Korea to those in the drought-stricken areas of Africa, India, and other places around the globe, they all have one thing in common: None of these countries are struggling with obesity or obesity related diseases simply because of the amount and types of food available in the environment in which they live. It doesn't matter what type of genes people are born with, if they are big-boned or thin-boned, or if they have a family history of being pre-disposed to obesity, when people live in an environment where food is scarce, no one is obese. While I'm in no way advocating starvation, I am suggesting that people make better choices. Just because one has unlimited access to food, this environment shouldn't dictate their eating habits to the extent where they become obese.

In fact, if one did happen to see an obese 500 or 600-pound obese person living amongst malnourished, starving people, it would surely make news head-lines around the world. Why can't the so called "fat gene" keep a person from losing weight in an environment where people are underweight due to the lack of food?

Shouldn't this gene interact with what little food they do consume and cause them to gain weight uncontrollably? According to many people who believe they struggle with this fat gene problem, it doesn't matter what they eat: they seem to spontaneously and magically gain weight.

I've heard some say that they hardly eat anything, yet they struggle with obesity on a daily basis. Recently, there was an interesting documentary about a man who weighed an astonishing 1250 pounds. He stated that he hardly ate anything and had absolutely no idea how he had managed to gain so much weight. Now I am quite sure, if this man was dropped off in some remote part of the world, where the food supply was very limited, he would actually be just as thin as other people living in the area, and not weighing more than half a ton.

Sometime later, after several interviews, it was determined that he had actually been eating quite a bit of food on a daily basis. An average breakfast consisted of 2 dozen eggs, 24 sausages and 6 boxes of cinnamon swirls (loaded with sweeteners like sugar, sugar invert, corn syrup, dextrose, maltodextrin, rice syrup and high fructose corn syrup), all eaten in just one setting. He had eaten himself to the point where he had become physically immobile and could not walk anymore. This condition exasperated his obesity problem, because he was consuming far too many calories than he was physically able to burn off.

Confined to his bed he had to helplessly and totally depend on someone else to prepare and bring his meals to him. Eventually, he had to be removed from his home with a crane used to weigh cattle. His overexposure to food had become such a health hazard it almost cost him his life. He was one week away from dying when medical intervention helped save his life. Upon arriving at the hospital, doctors immediately placed him on a special semi-liquid diet and restricted the amount of food he could consume daily. Amazingly, within 1 year, after weighing more than a half-ton, he had managed to lose 450 pounds; that's nearly one third of his previous body weight. He also managed to regain some limited mobility.

By simply restricting his access to food and caloric intake, along with a little exercise, he had the same results as those people living in underdeveloped third world countries. Though he didn't experience any type of physiological metamorphosis, his environment, as it relate, to food, was dramatically altered, and just like the people living in the underdeveloped countries, his body weight precipitously started falling off. It didn't matter if his fat gene was active or not. Once his environment changed – with regard to the amounts and types of fats, carbohydrates, calories, processed foods available to him – so did his weight. Again I'm not in any way trying to imply that there is something good about being poor and starving. I'm simply trying to make the point that having unlimited access to food is not always the best option for most people and can have ad- verse consequences.

Over the years, I have helped countless people manage their weight, including myself. I didn't give them nutritional information based on what type of genes they had. I simply had them change the types of foods they were used to eating, and had them incorporate some type of simple routine exercise regimen. Let me further explain away the fat gene theory and other fat-causing myths, with the following example:

The Dinka tribe, in the southern Sudan of Africa, practice a tradition passed down in their culture for centuries. Every year the men from the Dinka tribe take part in a competition that involves the participants gaining as much weight as possible within a certain time frame. Whoever gains the most weight wins a number of cattle, which increases his status in the tribe. The more cattle a man has, the wealthier he is considered to be, and the more wives he is allowed to marry and care for. In order to accomplish what would ordinarily seem impossible in a country where famine and starvation is commonplace (and where, of course, there are no overweight or obese people), the competitors are instructed to consume large quantities of fresh whole cow's milk daily, which is high in fat and protein. In addition to drinking lots of milk, these young men are also restricted from working and engaging in physical activity, basically forcing them into a sedentary lifestyle.

Every day until the competition ends, these men sit around and drink as much milk as possible. Their restricted movements require that they totally rely on others to milk the cows for them, and supply their daily rations. It is amazing to see their incredible transformation, as these men are able to gain an astonishing 60 to 70 pounds in a relatively short period of time. They simply add more milk to their diets and restrict almost all physical activity. During this annual competition, some of the men quickly gain too much weight, causing them to become ill and even die. Their small-framed bodies simply can't deal with the enormous amount of stress brought on by the dramatic and sudden change in weight.

However, it is a chance many of them are willing to take just to increase their prospects of gaining more wealth and status within the tribal community. The men supplying the milk never gain any weight; only those who are participating in the competition gain weight as they consume large quantities of fresh cows' milk. Here I noticed the only thing that changed was their environment as more milk was introduced into their daily dietary lifestyles. While normal milk intake and physical activity resulted in virtually no changes in tribal weight as a whole, those men who participated in the competition experienced well-documented weight gain. Drinking more milk than the average person in the tribe enabled these men to gain enormous amounts of weight, with some the men becoming obese in a relatively short period of time.

The other side of this story is just as amazing. After the competition ended, the men returned to their prior dietary habits and physical activity. Incredibly, these same men quickly lost the weight they had gained and returned back to their pre-competition sizes. Again, the only thing that changed as it related to their environment was the amount of milk they consumed daily and the return to normal physical activity. As the men drank less milk they all shared the same results, which was a dramatic drop in weight. Now, I used this example to clearly illustrate that it didn't matter what their genetic disposition may have been. All of their bodies responded to the sudden changes in diet, both in gaining weight and losing weight. In all these situations the results were the same: the less food made available to people in any environment, the less weight they are able to gain or maintain. As in the case of the Dinka Tribe, the greater amount of milk made available to them in their diets, the more weight they were able to gain and maintain, which was the ultimate purpose of the competition.

Obviously, I don't expect anyone to go out and starve themselves, because that would be unhealthy and cause severe adverse medical problems. So, how do people limit themselves in an environment where food is readily available 24 hours a day? Simply put, you would have to make a conscious decision and chose to make healthier food and beverage choices and limit intake of processed foods. Believe me, I love food too much to even consider starving myself, but I have managed to maintain my current weight for almost 30 years without dieting, counting calories, or watching fat intake. Genetically speaking, I should have had a hard time managing my weight because a lot of people in my family are over-weight. I was able to lose this "fat gene" or put it into remission by modifying my behavior as it related to nutrition and healthier lifestyle habits. The only thing that I have done differently over the past years is change how and what I eat and drink.

First, I drink water only as my main source of hydration. Secondly, even though I don't eat meat, I suggest eating carbohydrates and animal-based proteins separately. And thirdly, I began engaging in some type of aerobic and non-aerobic exercise at least three or more times weekly. Not only does all this help me to effortlessly maintain my weight, it also helps to build strong bones, healthy joints, and lean muscle mass. It's important to maintain lean muscle mass because it keeps your metabolism elevated, which helps the body burn more fat and calories even when you're resting. I have helped countless individuals reach their weight loss goals with this same approach. It didn't matter what types of genes they had or their family's predisposition to obesity they all experienced the same results. Some lost weight very quickly, while others lost weight more incrementally.

However, the outcome was still the same: a noticeable reduction in weight. I suppose the greatest benefit was that none of these people had to go on any type of diet. They simply modified their behavior regarding food, learned proper food combining techniques, and became more physically active. I also want to point out that some people lose weight without regular exercise. However, those who have the most success do incorporate some type of physical activity. It has been proven in study after study that people who are physically active live healthier and longer lives than those who are not. Leave the fat gene in the laboratory and start modifying your behavior by adopting healthier lifestyle habits. Habits such as eating less and engaging in more routine exercise will be far more advantageous to your weight loss strategy than trying to learn and figure out the latest "fat gene" theory.

STAYING FIT INCREASES YOUR FINANCIAL NET WORTH

CHAPTER VI

With the cost of living constantly on the rise these days, everyone could use a little extra cash. I'm quite sure while shopping lately for groceries you spent more money on common items such as milk, eggs, bread, poultry, fruit, and vegetables. With food being the largest expenditure of the average family's day-to-day budget, more than even the cost of gasoline, more and more families are feeling the squeeze on their pocketbooks.

Oh, and since I mentioned gasoline, I'm quite sure when leaving the grocery store you couldn't help but notice gas prices slowly creeping up as you stopped to refill your tank. We also have to pay more for movie tickets and dining out than ever before. Even utility bills are taking a larger chunk out of your paycheck every month. With college tuition, amusement park and airline tickets, shoes, and clothing all costing more, you may be wondering where you can get a much needed financial break.

Yes, everyone enjoys the benefit of having more money at their disposal. In fact, many people will go to great lengths just to get their hands on some extra spending cash. Some will work two jobs or countless hours of overtime in their pursuit of more income. Sadly, people waste billions annually, decreasing their net worth, by buying lottery tickets in hopes of hitting the jackpot. They gamble and take chances, hoping things will go in their favor, even though in most cases they only have a 1-in-55 million chance of winning. Talk about the odds being stacked against you!

According to researchers, the two primary things people are most pre-occupied with today is being wealthy and staying healthy. Well, you've probably never thought about it, but managing your weight and staying physically fit can put more dollars in your pocket than you might realize. By simply choosing to lose weight, you can instantly earn more money. That's right, you can actually increase your financial net worth, giving yourself the needed break you deserve just by watching your waistline—and it's all legal! While you can't control inflation or the fluctuations in interest rates, you can limit their impact by losing weight and staying physically fit. Scientists have finally made a direct correlation between our hunger for food and our hunger for fuel. They have discovered you can get better gas mileage by carrying less baggage, emptying your trunk, and yes, even losing weight. Here's a good example:

We are told gas prices in this country are controlled by decisions made by the OPEC cartel. Since none of us have any personal connection to this organization, we're not likely going to get any price breaks at the pumps. However, the leaner you are, the further you can travel on a tank of gas, which means you get more miles to the gallon. The more you weigh, the more fuel your car consumes, and the shorter distance you can travel. Here's another way of looking at it: Let's say you have four people traveling in an SUV, each of whom is 100 pounds or more overweight, which is not uncommon today. That's an additional 400 hundred pounds, and this extra weight will shorten the distance the SUV can travel.

Airlines know this best, as they have to pay more in extra fuel cost to fly heavier passengers. New research suggests that Americans are burning 1 billion more gallons of gasoline annually than they did in 1960 because of expanding waistlines. Research in the airline industry has proven overweight passengers contribute to higher fuel cost for the airline industry. With the average person being up to 30 pounds heavier than they were 40 years ago, it is estimated that more than 39 million gallons of fuel are used annually for every additional pound of passenger weight. That's enough extra fuel to fill roughly 2 million cars with gas for an entire year, and it can be directly attributed to expanding waistlines. This is just one example of the enormous financial benefits that staying in shape can have.

Now let's say, for example, your employer gives you a company car. You can actually increase the company's profitability by helping save on the cost of fuel if you are a leaner employee. If they give you a daily allowance for food your cost to eat would be lower too if you weighed less. Just imagine the savings we could accrue if every city employee like police officers, fire fighters, sanitation workers, bus drivers and government personnel decided to shed a few pounds. Who knows, with these extra savings, employers could consider returning the favor and give everybody a pay raise!

Here's another good example of how shrinking your waistline can make you wealthier: The smaller your waistline the cheaper your life insurance policy could be. One incentive used by insurance companies, considering the growing obesity epidemic in the United States, is to give customers discounts on their insurance premiums based on how well they are able to control their weight. One such insurance company, the Phoenix Company, is the first in the nation to offer this program. Customers who have written verification from their doctors, with a BMI (body mass index) in the range of 19-25 (standard size) receive a 20% discount on their life insurance policies. Insurance companies prize healthy customers because they live longer. They earn more revenues from physically fit customers who pay monthly premiums well into their 70s than from customers who die years earlier from natural causes. These companies look at your BMI because it has been statistically proven to be a good measure of longevity, which is one of their first considerations. And in fact, men and women who are in the normal BMI range actually do live longer.

These are just a few of the ways you can do your part to contribute to help lower the nation's overall health care cost. Your decision to incorporate the behavior modification techniques outlined in this book will help this generation and future generations to remain fit and healthy. So before you sit down to eat your next meal, take a moment to stop and think about how many people you can help. Imagine the impact you'd have! If you ever wanted to make a huge difference and positively impact another person's life, here is your opportunity. Not only are you helping other people, because everyone pays more in health care cost as a direct result of obesity and obesity related diseases, but you will also enhance your own health and your own wealth, enabling you to live longer without suffering from the devastating and debilitating complications associated with being overweight.

Speaking of diseases, I've compiled my own estimation of the costs to treat obesity and other related diseases, which impacts every tax payer in this country. Before I give these numbers, let me reiterate: Obesity is a preventable condition that is caused by bad eating habits and a sedentary lifestyle. Taxpayers foot the doctor's bill for more than half of obesity-related medical costs in this country via publicly funded Medicare and Medicaid programs, which cover sicknesses caused by obesity, including Type 2 diabetes, cardiovascular disease, gallbladder disease, and several types of cancers. The following numbers are an estimation of the total annual cost of obesity in the U.S.—though, keep in mind, the actual cost is probably higher than the figures I have listed:

<><><>

- The cost to treat heart disease: $8.8 billion
- Type 2 diabetes: $110 billion
- Osteoarthritis: $21.2 billion
- Hypertension: $4.1 billion
- Gallbladder disease: $3.4 billion
- Breast cancer: $2.9 billion
- Endometrial cancer: $933 million
- Colon cancer: $3.5 billion.

The total cost? $154 billion, and there's roughly another 22 or so diseases I didn't mention that are also directly related to obesity. I want you to look at these figures again and stop and think for a moment. Ask yourself if you are really doing all you can do to reduce your waistline and help lower this cost. Ask yourself, could I really get by drinking a six-pack of water instead of Diet Coke? Could I eat a couple of apples instead of a box of Little Debbie's snack cakes?

I think if you were to really be honest with yourself, you could easily come up with the correct answers. If you want to give it a shot, this book will help you by teaching you behavior modification techniques that can make a difference. Just think, you will never have to diet again, and you can keep the weight off permanently. We all need your help and we're all counting on you to help make the difference. This nation could save $5.6 billion annually in costs associated with treating heart disease alone, if just one-tenth of Americans began walking regularly. We would save another $100 billion if people adopted healthier nutritional habits, exercised routinely, and reduced their consumption of junk food. With these savings alone, it is easy to see how everyone around you benefits when you are in good health. Every taxpayer, employer. state agency, local government agency, community, your family, your friends, and the entire country gains when you lose weight because it lowers the overall cost of health care for everyone.

That's right, you can be the skinniest person in America and someone else's waistline will impact you financially. And as I have previously stated, the financial rewards gained from slimming down don't just benefit this current generation, but the next one as well. Learning how to apply and teach the behavior modification techniques found in this book creates instant wealth. Staying healthy and fit is not just about financial gains; it's also about physical and psychological rewards. You feel more confident about yourself when you are in shape. You also relieve yourself of the constant mental anguish and stress of having to worry about others teasing or ostracizing you because of your weight.

Losing weight is one of the easiest ways to improve your economic competitiveness, especially in the work place. By reducing your waistline you become a more valuable asset to your employer, instead of a financial liability or risk. It has been proven that overweight and obese individuals are more likely to file workers' compensation claims for injuries on the job. Researchers were able to confirm a significant association between BMI and on-the job back, wrist, neck, shoulder, knee, foot and hip injuries. Additional research suggests older Americans who are overweight may have a higher risk of disability. Obesity is an increasing public health problem, and a risk factor for many chronic diseases and premature death.

Those with the highest BMIs (40 and over) have twice the rate of workers' compensation claims than those at the recommended weight. This adds to the number of lost work days, as the cost per claim increases rapidly. Researchers have found that the number of lost days for obese employees was 13 times higher compared to those of regular weight. Although many types of injury are associated with high BMI, researchers have found a more pronounced relationship between was high BMI and inflammation, contusions, and strains. Given the strong effect of BMI on work injuries, it's not only important for workers to maintain healthy weight, but it should also be a high priority for employers as well.

Along with companies stressing workplace safety, healthy eating and physical activity should be emphasized as well.

Years ago one could count on a college degree to help them advance in their career objectives however that's no longer the case. Today, having a poor BMI might adversely affect your ability to compete for certain jobs. More and more research points to a direct correlation between this number and loss of worker productivity. Overweight employees mean more time off and fewer worker production hours.

The Centers for Disease Control and Prevention defines obesity as a BMI of 30 or more; people between 25 and 30 are considered overweight; those in the range of 19 to 25 are considered normal weight. A higher BMI equates to higher insurance premiums, hospital bills, and prescription medication cost. You really can't blame employers for being selective; they have to watch their bottom line or the corporation may not be profitable. Today, many employers are offering cash incentives to employees who either lose weight or manage their current weight. Two major corporations, Dow Chemical and Home Depot, have teamed up with major universities and the National Institute of Health to develop environmental interventions to help people manage their diet and weight. The National Business Group on Health, a Washington, D.C.-based, non-profit organization that represents large companies, recently gathered the following statistics:

$93 billion of the nation's medical bills are directly related to treating obesity and other conditions related to overweight conditions. Corporate America covers $14 billion of this cost, which includes $1.5 billion for disability insurance, another $10 billion for health insurance and paid sick leave, and almost $2 billion for life insurance.

The economic cost of workplace obesity translates into 239 million days annually where work activity is restricted, 90 million sick days or days in bed, 63 million visits to physicians, and 39 million lost work days. The Los Angeles County Sheriff's Department recently announced a hiring freeze on prospective candidates that did not meet the department's newly revised weight guidelines. They understand the negative impact excessive weight can have on an officer's performance in the field.

We have all been entertained by late night TV personalities and their jokes about the love affair between police officers and donut shops. Believe it or not, there is a pound or more of truth to those jokes. Consumption of these sweet and fattening delicacies can definitely lead to weight gain, as most are fried in hydrogenated oil, which is even worse for your waistline than eating lard. In my opinion if you are going to eat donuts, you should definitely do some type of high impact cardiovascular workout and drink plenty of water before and after. Today, with many jobs being performance-based, losing weight dramatically helps to improve your economic competitiveness. For example people who sit at computers all day are more inclined to be overweight, and therefore cost more to employ. Put yourself in your boss's shoes for a moment and consider if you had someone working for you. In such a situation, you would naturally want them to be an asset to your company and not a liability. Well, your boss is no different. Many employers require that you stay within certain weight limits in order to maintain your salary or receive a promotion. They really don't have a choice because statistically overweight employees file more workers compensation claims.

This extra liability causes employers to be a bit more selective about whom they choose to hire. Many other government agencies are starting to feel the impact obesity is having on job performance. Police officers are probably affected even more so, because they have to chase an endless supply of bad guys, who normally work out as part of their trade. Having to chase someone down when you are out of shape can be a real health hazard, and can lead to higher incidents of work-related injuries. Some of these injuries can be permanent or even result in life-threatening complications. In addition, when you're overweight, the person being pursued has a higher probability of getting away, which could result in an increased danger to the general public.

Lastly, researchers have discovered that your ZIP code could actually say a whole lot more about you than what state or city you live in. For most of our lives, we have associated ZIP codes as a way to send and receive mail. However, recent studies reveal that ZIP codes in areas with the highest residential property values had the slimmest residents. I was surprised to learn that the lower the home values happened to be in a particular ZIP code, the higher the incidence of obesity there was amongst the residents. In some of the lowest assessed residential areas, the obesity rate was as high as 30%.

Because higher BMIs are associated with increased worker's compensation claims, in the future, where you live could seriously jeopardize your chances of landing that next job, especially if the company uses your ZIP code as a gage for employment in the same way they now use BMI measurements. This new revelation regarding the relationship between obesity and ZIP codes could really blow away the theories circulating about obesity being caused by genetic factors. Look, for instance, at wealthy states like New Hampshire, Rhode Island, Massachusetts, and Maine, which all have lower rates of obesity. Now turn your attention to states in the south like Mississippi, Alabama, Louisiana, and West Virginia, all of which have the highest rates of obesity in the country.

Take a ZIP code like 90210 in Beverly Hills, California, and then take a ZIP code like 90062 in South Central Los Angeles. There is a huge disparity between these two zip codes as residents in South Central have a disproportionately higher obesity rate. Thus, obesity has more to do with social economic status than any genetic factors. In regards to the wealthy and poor geographical areas, I would hope that no one in their right mind would even insinuate that only people with fat-free genes live in the wealthier states, while those with fat genes live in poor southern states.

In support of these findings" City Councilwoman Jan Perry proposed a moratorium on fast food restaurants in the poverty-stricken areas of South Central Los Angeles. The proposed ordinance would stop new fast-food restaurants from opening in the area for up to 2 years while the city establishes a long-term plan to deal with the restaurants that have been linked to health problems. This is a response to suspicions that obesity and other related illnesses including high blood pressure, diabetes, and heart disease are connected to the high-fat foods that dominate fast food restaurant menus in lower socioeconomic areas like South Central Los Angeles.

Research suggests South Central Los Angeles has the county's highest concentration of fast food restaurants. The area also has higher rates of obesity than the rest of the county, with 30% of adults being obese, compared with 20.9% in the county overall. For children, the obesity rate was 29% in South Central Los Angeles, compared with 23.3% nationwide. The study reveals significant geographic disparity in the obesity problem, which is very much related to socio-economic status and dietary lifestyle. The nature of the neighborhood determines access to healthy foods. Organic supermarket chain such as Trader Joe's, for example, is situated across the country in areas where the greatest buying power is from universities and affluent neighborhoods. Unfortunately, people living in impoverished neighborhoods are relegated in some cases to buying their groceries at gas stations and eating mostly high-fat, sodium rich fast foods.

Research shows that obese parents are more likely to have obese children, and some children will suffer the same obesity-related illnesses as their parents. So, as you can easily see, the overall cost to an employer in insurance premiums for an entire family that is overweight can be staggering over time. Without profits, no company can operate a viable successful business. It was once reported that General Motors spent more money to pay for obesity-related health care costs than they did to buy steel used to build cars.

One reason we have seen a dramatic increase in the number of companies out-sourcing American jobs to other countries is due to higher health care cost associated with employee illnesses, which to some extent is directly related to overweight and obese employees in this country. These companies are under tremendous pressure to stay competitive in their perspective industries. To accomplish this, they must have a workforce that is healthier than their competitors. Once more before we close the chapter, let's go over the benefits of losing weight and staying fit:

You: increase your economic competitiveness and become a better employment prospect; receive discounts on insurance premiums; spend less on groceries, clothing, fuel for your car and dining out; have fewer doctor visits and insurance co-pays; stay more mobile; prevent chronic diseases; have less expenses associated with prescription medications; have fewer hospital visits; lower worker's compensation claims; become a greater financial asset to your employer and less of a burden to your family and friends; suffer fewer illnesses; and prevent diabetes, hypertension, heart disease, joint problems, certain forms of cancer, Obesity-related depression and sleep apnea. By losing weight you save everyone in the country, your family, neighbors, friends, the government, and your unborn offspring a lot of money. With all the negative complications associated with excessive weight, why not stay fit? It's definitely to your advantage as well.

OBESITY AND MEDICAL INTERVENTION

CHAPTER VII

$\mathcal{A}$s the number of obese people continues to steadily rise with no effective remedy in sight, medical intervention is quickly becoming a very popular way to battle bulging waste lines. Today, almost half of this nation's adult population and children are obese, with the morbidly obese now the fastest growing section of this country's population. Thanks to Hollywood role models, everyone wants to sport that "perfect ten" body, or get as close to it as possible. It seems no matter what the cost or unknown health risk associated with these medical procedures, many don't care and just want to be thin, sexy, and beautiful. Even our young people have jumped on the band wagon as obesity surgeries among teens have more than tripled in recent years.

There are three popular medical weight loss procedures commonly performed here in the U.S. They can range in price anywhere from a couple thousand dollars up to $35,000. These medical procedures consist of gastric bypass surgery, liposuction, and lipolysis. All these surgical options have reported side effects, with gastric bypass and liposuction the most costly and painful. These procedures are all relatively new, as compared to regular dieting, and, according to the latest research, are totally ineffective as well. People should be fully aware and clearly understand that medical intervention will not cause you to lose weight permanently, nor help you manage your weight.

After the cutting, slicing, suctioning, and injections, it is still up to each individual patient to practice healthier lifestyle habits. In fact, without incorporating healthier behavior modification techniques, patients generally regain the weight they've lost. I can tell you now this book is cheaper and less painful than any medical procedure and carries no adverse side effects. People who spend $35,000 to get most of their stomach and intestines removed have to use these same techniques after surgery in order to ensure the procedure is successful. As I stated before and will continue to stress, no amount of dieting, weight loss pills or medical intervention can replace, nor can they be an alternative to, healthy life-style changes.

The first procedure is called lipolysis where patients are injected with a chemical substance that dissolves fat. It's the cheapest and is designed for those who only have a very small area of excess fat they are trying to remove. Because it is a non-invasive, non-surgical, relatively simple procedure, and only costs around $2,000, it is becoming increasingly popular. The procedure involves a patient receiving between 5-25 treatments spread out over a period of 2-4 weeks. Patients normally receive injections in their neck, thighs, bellies, upper arms, and other fatty areas they want to shrink. The best treatment areas are said to be the abdomen, flanks, and under the chin. Disfiguring masses, infections, inflamed tissue, tissue death and allergic reactions have all been reported. In one particular case, a young lady's allergic reaction was so violent she had to be admitted to the hospital emergency ward where she was covered in hives from head to toe. Recently, the American Society for Aesthetic Plastic Surgery issued a warning against the use of injections for fat-loss treatments. Also, this procedure has not yet been approved by the FDA.

Phosphatidylcholine, one of the ingredients in lipodissolve injections, is derived from soybean oil and deoxycholatem, a bile salt. They are mixed together and cause an inflammatory response in the body that breaks open and destroys fat cells. Supposedly, the broken down materials are carried to the liver, processed, and then excreted harmlessly out of the body. However, critics argue this process hasn't been scientifically proven and it isn't clear where the dissolved fat goes. It may be filtered out by the liver or kidneys, or deposited in the blood vessels. If it's dumped into the blood vessels, it can very easily turn into potentially damaging unstable molecules called "free radicals." These free radicals constantly circulating in the blood can lead to heart disease and/or sudden death syndrome.

Many experts contend that more peer-reviewed studies need to be conducted to discuss the safety and efficiency of lipodissolve. Again, this procedure will not remove pounds of fat, but rather inches in small areas. In the end, the results will not be permanent unless you modify your behavior and practice healthier lifestyle habits. The next medical procedure, known as liposuction, it involves doctors using a vacuuming device to literally suck fat from the body. The procedure can cost up to $10,000 and can be very painful, often requiring several weeks of recovery time. Liposuction is said to permanently remove fat cells, however this is not totally true. The body produces fat cells as needed, and these cells are then stored in various areas of the body.

The naturally balanced 80/20 ratio of subcutaneous to visceral fat storage ensures that too much fat does not collect in vital areas where it can become disruptive and harmful. The major problem with liposuction is that the permanent removal of fat cells in one area could permanently alter this delicate balance, causing new fat cells to relocate in other areas of the body. If it collects around the liver, heart, or pancreas, this could lead to deadly degenerative diseases. Also, there is little blood circulation around fat, which equals less available oxygen. This environment is perfect for the proliferation of disease-causing pathogens, viruses and bacteria. So while people may want to manipulate certain areas of their body to give it a much healthier and sexier appearance, they could actually be setting themselves up for some disastrous health consequences down the road.

Again, as with lipolysis, following liposuction you still have to practice healthier lifestyle habits or you will end up gaining weight all over again. Again the procedure does not create permanent weight loss, because the body will continue to make new fat cells when necessary. The body manufactures fat perpetually from the food you eat and if it isn't immediately used for energy, it is stored away for future use. Last but not least, the most drastic, invasive, and life-changing medical procedure, which I call the "granddaddy of them all," is gastric bypass surgery. The focus of this surgery is to force a person to take in fewer calories by dramatically reducing the size of their stomach. With a smaller stomach and eating smaller portions, fewer calories are consumed, so a person will be able to lose weight and keep it off.

Gastric bypass surgery may be popular, but it doesn't come without a hefty physical toll on the body. It is a permanent and irreversible procedure that requires permanent and irreversible lifestyle changes as well. There have been numerous reported cases of people suffering adversely after undergoing this procedure, with some reported deaths as well. No one knows the long-term health risks associated with gastric bypass surgery. According to all the available research and expert opinions, this kind of surgery is so new we will just have to wait to see what the future reveals.

Fortunately, the operation is normally restricted to exceedingly obese people who are more than 100 pounds overweight. These patients often have medical problems as a result of being obese, including heart disease, diabetes, and respiratory problems. Sometimes gastric surgery can alleviate these problems, but the conditions can also contribute to making the surgery more risky. A patient qualifies for the surgery if all other attempts at losing weight have previously failed. The procedure is very painful and expensive, costing around $35,000 per operation, including hospital stays, and is not covered by Medicare unless the obesity is contributing to other health issues.

Obesity experts have recommended that Medicare not pay for this type of procedure because it is not an effective solution to long-term permanent weight loss. These experts contend that regardless of what type of medical surgery is performed, the patients fail to acknowledge an inescapable reality. Unless people are willing to incorporate healthier behavior modification techniques such as eating habits and exercise, no surgery can give lasting successful results. With obesity surgery fast becoming a popular way to battle the nation's weight crisis, it may actually be a lot riskier than most people understand. New research has revealed some unsettling revelations about the higher-than-expected risk of death in the year after surgery, even among teen patients.

Dr. David Flum, a surgeon at the University of Washington and lead author of a Medicare study that analyzed this risk, says the deaths are a wake-up call for those considering this operation. In previous studies the reported death rate was under 1% for people in their 30s to their 50s, which are the most common ages for gastric bypass surgery. However, in a new Medicare study of 16,155 patients who had the procedure, more than 5% of men and nearly 3% of women in this age group were dead within a year, although the percentage of death a year after surgery amongst those aged 45-54 were slightly higher.

There are several different types of gastric bypass procedure to choose from. The most common operation normally involves surgical shrinking of the stomach. The surgery's potentially deadly complications can include malnutrition, infection coupled with bowel and gallbladder problems. In older patients especially, any type of drastic surgery of this type can be a deadly shock to the system. Despite the health risks involved, gastric bypass surgery has increased more than ten-fold since 1998, which parallels the surge in the rate of obese people in this country.

Gastric bypass involves creating an egg-size pouch in the upper stomach and attaching it to a section of intestine. Doctors who perform the operation normally remove 90% of the stomach and 75% of the small intestines. I want to reiterate here that after having the procedure, a patient still has to permanently practice healthy behavior modification techniques or the surgery will be a complete failure.

The surgery in and of itself won't cause a person to lose weight; it simply prepares them for the dietary changes they will have to make to accomplish permanent weight loss. Ultimately, it is up to each individual patient to make the necessary changes and modify his or her behavior as it relates to proper nutrition, hydration, and exercise. I have listed several side effects that may occur as a result of gastric bypass. Because so much of the stomach and intestines are removed during this operation, a patient will lack enzymes, digestive juices, and stomach acids, which are used to liquefy food and prepare it for further digestion. This will permanently cause improper digestion and nutrient assimilation, resulting in malnutrition.

Because of this, patients will have to commit to taking vitamins, minerals, and some protein supplements for the rest of their lives or risk becoming very ill. The cost for these supplies will run from $600-1,200 annually, depending on the quality of the supplements purchased. The newly designed stomach pouch will make patients uncomfortable if they eat too much or eat too fast, which can cause vomiting. Bypassing the duodenum can cause metabolic bone disease in some patients, resulting in bone pain, loss of height, humped back, and rib and hipbone fractures. Additional adverse side effects include chronic anemia, diarrhea, hair loss, nutritional deficiencies, some loss of absorptive function, gallstones, mood changes, fatigue, flu-like symptoms, and deficiencies in certain vitamins and minerals, especially vitamin B-12, iron, calcium and folate.

Another adverse side effect some patients may experience is known as "dumping syndrome" as a result of eating too much sugar or too much food. Symptoms can include faintness, sweating, weakness, vomiting, nausea, and occasionally diarrhea. In fact, some patients are no longer able to tolerate sugary or oily foods after undergoing this procedure. Poor absorption of iron and calcium can cause low total body iron and a greater chance of contracting iron deficiency anemia.

A few years ago, I met a young lady in her early 20s who had gone through this procedure. She was suffering with quite a few of the permanent side effects associated with the surgery. She explained to me that she had a difficult time digesting oily foods and that they made her feel nauseous. She had to totally modify her diet and lifestyle to accommodate the new changes as a result of the surgery. Just like this young lady, all gastric bypass patients will have to closely and carefully monitor what types of foods they consume after the operation. With 90% of their stomach missing, they will be limited to eating only very small portions. A large portion of their meals will have to be liquefied and certain types of fats will have to be eliminated. Furthermore, a full 10% of patients don't lose any weight at all; doctors believe these patients have somehow figured out a way to cheat and consume more calories without getting sick.

After the procedure, patients are advised to adjust their lifestyle in the following three areas:

1) Nutrition: Patients are advised to stop eating when they feel full, even if it seems as if they haven't eaten enough. Overeating by just one bite may cause significant discomfort, including vomiting. Patients will no longer need a lot of food and should take very small bites of whatever they eat, making sure to chew their food well and slowly, with a normal meal lasting about 30 minutes to an hour to consume. In addition, they will have to eat foods they can tolerate and avoid high-calorie dishes.

2) Hydration: Patients are advised not to drink liquids with their meals, but instead drink 30 minutes prior to or an hour after meals. Drinking during the meal will cause a sensation of pressure in the chest that is uncomfortable and can cause the food to back up. Between meals, it is advisable to drink 4-to-6 glasses of water to maintain optimum fluid intake. Liquids that are high in calories should be avoided, because taking in extra calories between meals

will result in slower weight loss, and patients will not achieve the weight they desire.

3) Exercise: A regular exercise program is vital and highly recommended while recovering from any gastric bypass surgery procedure. Walking is one of the most effective forms of exercise for this purpose. Patients are advised to start with very short walks several times a day and gradually increase the distance. Even with exercise, patients fail to experience significant weight loss, primarily because they persist in consuming high calorie liquids or soft foods, such as peanut butter, ice cream, and sodas, which readily slide through the little stomach pouch.

Professionals in this field stress that the surgery in and of itself will not miraculously cure obesity, and the best results are obtained when patients practice good dietary and exercise habits. In other words, those who fail to adjust end up regaining their weight, putting their health at risk and wasting $35,000. In the previous chapter, I intentionally highlighted three key strategic areas of behavior modification techniques you will find repeatedly stressed throughout this book. They are: proper nutrition, hydration, and exercise.

In fact, obesity specialists stress that with every approach to losing weight such as dieting, diet pills, and medical intervention, a person has to practice healthier behavior modification techniques in order to have a successful outcome. These same professionals also maintain the idea that regardless of which method is used studies show the same inescapable reality: No surgery gives lasting results unless people also change eating and exercising habits.

Which brings us right back to why I wrote this book in the first place; learning behavior modification techniques as a preventative tool to avoid ever having the need for any of these procedures is the safest and best approach. It would be more beneficial to invest your hard earned money into something more profitable for yourself and your family, such as a retirement account or your child's college fund. Ultimately, patients who do not adopt healthier lifestyle habits end up gaining back their weight and becoming another sad statistic.

REVERSING CHILDHOOD OBESITY

CHAPTER VIII

*I*t's time for World leaders to sign an executive order declaring childhood obesity a global emergency. The obesity rate among our young people has spiraled dangerously out of control, affecting nearly half of all children in United States. The Center for Disease Control is reporting that obesity rates have nearly quintupled among youth between the ages of 6 and 11. It further concluded children between 2 and 5 years of age, as well as teenagers, have seen a threefold increase in weight in the past 30 years.

The medical consequences of obesity-related diseases like diabetes, high cholesterol, hypertension, and orthopedic problems are costing this country more than $100 billion annually. More frightening is the fact that 30 years ago, these diseases were rarely seen amongst younger people. When I was growing up, I had never heard of or witnessed other young people my age suffering from diabetes or heart disease. Forgive me, but I'll be reiterating throughout this entire book the fact that obesity is a preventable disease resulting from poor nutritional habits and a sedentary lifestyle. People are choosing, either knowingly or unknowingly, to practice unhealthy eating and lifestyle habits.

Sadly, as I pen this book, 1 out of every 3 children in this country is over-weight, with Puerto Rico having the highest number of obese children hovering right around 26%. Walter Rivera-Saez, Puerto Rico's assistant secretary of health, has stated that if nothing is done to immediately reverse this trend, the current generation of Puerto Rican children will be the first to die before their parents from complications associated with diseases directly related to obesity.

Under the direction of Puerto Rico's governor Luis G. Fortuño, an $8 million program was launched called "Puerto Rico in Shape." In the program physical trainers and nutritionists were hired in each city to teach people about healthier nutrition and exercise.

Meanwhile, governor Fortuño has issued an executive order declaring childhood obesity an island-wide emergency.

One problem in Puerto Rican culture which is also common in other cultures, is a mind-set that actually celebrates pudginess in children as a sign of good health. However, scientific research suggests just the opposite and contends that over-weight children normally grow into overweight teens and eventually into over-weight adults. Chile and Mexico are two Latin American countries with obesity rates comparable to Puerto Rico. Some leaders have attacked the obesity epidemic head-on by eliminating many fatty foods from the school cafeterias. Brazil, like some states in the U.S., has banned soda from school vending machines.

While these are very positive changes, most of the vending machines are still stocked with obesity causing-substances. The culprits are fruity drinks and water sweetened with high fructose corn syrup, which is just as bad as, or in some cases worse than regular soda. Today, schools in states all across this country are trying to tackle the daunting task of reversing childhood obesity as part of a new government mandate. They are receiving a lot of help from state and federal government programs that are designed to help reduce obesity.

As parents, you probably already know how challenging it can be to get your children to eat more fruits and vegetables, if any at all. It's not difficult to understand why when you consider all the junk food commercials our children are bombarded with. It is estimated that children between the ages of 8 and 12 see an average of 21 television ads each day selling fast foods, cereals, snacks and candy. That is more than 7,600 commercials per year, according to a recent Kaiser Family Foundation study. What's even more amazing is that not one of the 8,854 ads reviewed in the Kaiser study promoted fruits or vegetables. The constant onslaught of advertising for unhealthy food products directly counters the values we as parents are trying to instill in our children about good nutritional behavior.

This situation is further complicated by the incredible availability of junk foods that counter sound nutritional education. Children have a keen awareness of junk food. It comes from every direction by way of commercials, stores, cartoons, comic books, and highway billboards. This relentless advertising is a major factor influencing what we constantly battle as parents. Making matters worse, many of these foods are heavily laden with as many as four different sweeteners, with high-fructose corn syrup at the top of the ingredient list. This brings me to my next point. Sadly, most food conglomerates care more about keeping their shareholders happy than your child's health. Since this dangerous sweetener is dirt cheap, it saves these corporations lots of money, which they can spend on more advertising to our children.

Hopefully, you are as proactive as I am about your child's health. You must be steadfast and practical in taking the necessary steps to protect your child and ensure they are getting adequate and wholesome nutrition. If these major food conglomerates aren't going to take the necessary steps and start using better quality and healthier ingredients, then ultimately you as a parent will have to take matters into your own hands. It seems as if money is the primary motivating factor that can push these companies in the right direction. When they experience sluggish sales as a result of fewer junk food purchases, then they will get the message and take notice.

Let me prove my point here and you'll see how the power of money can change the mindset of top executives: Currently, two major children's cereal makers are in the process of changing the way they market their products to children. These companies say they are committed to increasing the nutritional value of cereals and snacks for kids. However, the change came only after parents and advocacy groups who were worried about obesity threatened a lawsuit. David Mackay, president and CEO of Kellogg's, said the company was taking action because of increasing concerns about marketing to children. As I said before, money talks, and the intense pressure from parents even brought about changes in the way these companies use images of foods in computer games, downloads, and wallpaper.

This is just a start, because more action is needed. Until then, the responsibility lies with us as good parents to guard the health of our children. I'll use my 6-year-old daughter as an example. Like most children her age, she loves eating starchy foods like noodles and macaroni and cheese. For years I tried searching for healthy alternatives she could eat, without any success. Every time we went to the grocery store, she would beg me to buy her just one more package of Top Ramen noodles.

I can vividly remember her saying, "Daddy, could you please buy me just one more package of Oodles of Noodles, and I promise never to ask for any more!" Even though I tried being firm with her, sometimes I couldn't resist her pleas and totally gave in. Then one day, I got an idea and decided to try something different. I prepared her a bowl of organic whole-wheat multi-grain noodles seasoned with organic butter and Celtic sea salt. To my surprise it was an instant hit and she even asked for seconds. Today, she loves the whole-wheat pasta, and the transition to the healthier choice was fairly easy.

After I sat down with her and explained the benefits of eating whole-wheat noodles versus the health risk associated with the highly refined noodles, she had no problem switching over to the whole-wheat pasta, and now actually requests it on a daily basis. The extra 5 minutes it took for me to prepare her noodles was well worth the peace of mind I got out of knowing she was eating a healthier meal. Currently, I am working on incorporating vegetables into her noodles, taking things slowly and moving one step at a time.

Another example is when she wants to eat at McDonalds. Instead of allowing her to get the normal hamburger, French fry, and soft drink combination, I will order her two hamburgers with water instead, with no fries or soft drink. This prevents the improper combining of a high-fat animal protein with a high-glycemic starch and a high fructose corn syrup-based beverage. This unhealthy combination will not digest properly and causes an enormous amount of glucose to be dumped into the blood. Again, excess glucose requires more insulin, which ultimately could lead to the pancreas being overworked. In this state the body also creates more fat cells, leading to unwanted weight gain. I sat down with my daughter and explained to her the risk associated with eating these types of meals, and just like the times before, she responded positively.

It has been my experience that convincing children to reverse bad habits is a much easier task than trying to convince adults. Many experts believe that reaching children before they hit puberty is essential in order to improve their eating habits. When children understand the health risk associated with these foods, I find that almost all of them have a genuine desire to change their eating habits. And this brings me to my next point. It is imperative that parents become more educated about what they are feeding their children and how unhealthy foods can actually endanger their children's health. Children can't be held responsible because they do not do the grocery shopping. If Mom is loading up the shopping cart with Oreo cookies, Cheetos, white bread, refined carbohydrates, and sugary drinks, then that's exactly what the child is going to eat.

If you are not proactive early on and your child does happen to become overweight, it is likely that they'll eventually resort to dieting. According to many experts, the last thing you should ever want is for your child to go on a diet. Recently, researchers at the University of Minnesota in Minneapolis discovered that teens who go on diets to lose weight will more than likely skip breakfast and binge eat, which could be part of the reason why they gain more weight over time than their peers who don't diet. These researchers further stated that people who are at a greater risk of becoming overweight are also more likely to have tried dieting in the past. The study entitled, Slimming Down Sets the Stage for Poor Eating Habits, stresses that most teens choose dieting, a short term fix, over behavior modification techniques that produce permanent long-term results.

Another study suggested that teenagers who are overweight are likely to have fewer children in adulthood. It also it revealed that obese teenagers were less likely than their normal-weight peers to live with a partner as an adult. The researchers suggested the growing global obesity pandemic could have wide-spread effects on adults' reproductive health. The study stated that obesity is related to reproductive difficulties and raises the risk of a number of other pregnancy complications. Men and women who were obese as teens are almost 38% more likely to have fewer children. In both women and men, obesity can lead to infertility problems. For example, a woman can become infertile from a disease called polycystic ovary syndrome. An obese man can experience lower sperm count as well as erectile dysfunction.

The results of their research stressed the potential long-term effects of obesity at a young age, offering one more reason why as parents we need to become proactive about helping prevent our children from having to resort to dieting in order to lose weight. Another area of concern should be the dramatic increase in the number of obese teens opting to have gastric bypass surgery. The number of U.S. children receiving obesity surgery has tripled in recent years. As previously mentioned the long-term adverse health consequences of this surgery are unknown at this point and could prove to be disastrous. Teens who have had the surgery say it is very painful, and ultimately they still end up having to adjust their diets. This book is designed to be used as a preventive tool, helping to educate people on how to use healthier behavioral modification techniques before gastric bypass is ever needed. Fortunately, this procedure is only offered as a last resort for most obese teens. Also, for many teens who already struggle with identity issues, experiencing rapid weight loss after surgery can catapult them into situations they didn't even imagine before.

Unfortunately, children living in poverty-stricken areas of this country are especially at risk for becoming overweight because unhealthy food is cheaper and more easily available than healthy food. Their parents are often single moms who sometimes have to leave their children unsupervised to get their own snacks. This problem is further exacerbated in low-income neighborhoods, where there are fewer healthy grocery stores with fresh produce, and a plethora of unhealthy fast-food restaurants serving fattening foods. If people don't have healthy options available to them, they can't make healthier choices. Another problem is most of these low socioeconomic status areas are gang-infested, causing many parents to fear for their children's lives. Children are forced to stay indoors, resulting in an involuntary sedentary lifestyle.

With teens, money makes a big difference in access to healthy diet and exercise. Researchers have discovered that those living in poverty have grown fatter at a higher rate than their more affluent peers. This revelation further underscores the unequal burden obesity places on the nation's impoverished residents. The percentage of overweight adolescents is about 50% higher in poor families as compared to wealthier families. Obesity rates climbed substantially among all teens during the past 30 years. But the great divide according to income was relatively unknown until recently. Yet, in my opinion, poverty is no excuse for obesity because it still boils down to healthy lifestyle habits. In truth, a bag of apples costs just as much as a bag of Oreo cookies, and a gallon of water is cheaper than a 3-liter bottle of soda.

In the early 1970s, about 4% of impoverished youngsters between the ages of 15 and 17 were severely overweight, compared with approximately 5% of teens who were not poor. In contrast, by the early 2000s, those rates leaped to 23% of the poor and 14% of other kids. This doesn't mean that the wealthy aren't getting fatter as well, because adult obesity rates have climbed the fastest in recent de-cades among those who earn more than $60,000 annually. Over the past decade the percentage of calories ingested from high-fructose corn syrup has grown by more than 20% among kids in the 15-17-year age range. Combine these unhealthy empty calories with little or no exercise, and a higher probability of adolescents who skip breakfast, and you have a disaster waiting to happen.

Since people who are overweight are at an increased risk for diabetes, heart disease, hypertension, joint problems, and other chronic conditions that contribute to higher health care costs, it is essential that we influence our children by exemplifying healthier lifestyle habits ourselves. This involves practicing healthy behavior techniques like consuming less junk food, eating more fruits and vegetables, and becoming more physically active. All of the medical research clearly demonstrates that these small changes can prevent not only obesity but also degenerative diseases as well. As parents, we must remain vigilant and reclaim the health of our children so they can live healthier, wealthier, and happier lives. Obese children experience more physical stress on their small-framed bodies than obese adults. They face a lot of peer pressure, and desperately want to be accepted by their peers. Over-weight children are often teased and harassed in school and social gatherings; they're usually chosen last when playing sports and singled out in other ways as well. Most adults who were obese as children have very bad memories about their childhood experiences.

Obesity poses a greater health risk to children than it does to adults. One reason for this is their little bodies are still growing. Doctors are warning obese 6-year-olds, who develop childhood hypertension and diabetes in their teens, could suffer fatal consequences from complications associated with these diseases by the time they reach their 40s. Unlike adults who get these diseases later in life after they have fully matured and live for a longer period of time, children are still growing and their bodies simply can't handle the stress brought to bear on them by degenerative diseases so early in their lives.

Fortunately it is not too late, because behavior modification techniques involving healthier nutrition and physical activity is the best way to reverse, manage, and prevent these diseases. There are numerous government-funded programs currently being offered that are designed to help both children and their parents. One such program based in Dallas is called LEAN (Lifestyle, Exercise and Nutrition). This program focuses on making fitness and nutritional changes for the whole family. The ultimate goal of the program is to teach families skills they can use for the rest of their lives. One family in the program reportedly went from eating fast food and sugary drinks for dinner to having grilled chicken, vegetables, and diet soda. I still recommend water over diet drinks because most of them contain some type of artificial sweetener that adversely affects the function of the liver.

Also, the best time to have a sweetened drink is 30 minutes to an hour prior to working out. This will produce an extra burst of energy and cleanse the blood of excess glucose so that insulin levels remain normal. I mention this because many experts believe exercise is the secret to slimmer kids. They say just 15-minute bursts of intense play might be enough to keep children from becoming over-weight. Exercises like swimming, soccer, brisk walking, and sprinting are the most effective at burning away deposits of visceral fat that normally surrounds the major organs, possibly preventing them from functioning properly.

Researchers in the U.S. and Britain found that children who did 15 minutes a day of moderate exercise were 50% less likely than inactive children to become obese. They stressed that higher-intensity physical activity may be more important than total activity. This study provides some of the first robust evidence on the link between physical activity and obesity in children. The great part is it only takes small amounts of effort to get dramatic results. Eating more calories than you are able to burn off will definitely trigger the onset of obesity. The less children exercise, the more likely they'll become obese. Even committing to 15 minutes of moderate and vigorous physical activity daily might result in an important reduction in the prevalence of obesity.

One final area to explore is the federally funded public school lunch programs, where it can be all too easy for your child to eat chicken nuggets, French fries, and other junk foods. In truth, it costs the same amount of money for schools to feed organic foods to children as it does non-organic foods. Again, getting the schools to serve healthier meals is where parent advocacy groups can have a huge impact. The food currently served in school cafeterias is of poor nutritional value, if it contains any nutrition at all. This is one reason why I recommend all parents supplement their child's diet with a high quality food-based organic multivitamin, mineral, and phytonutrient supplement.

The poor quality of your child's school lunch is another reason why as parents we should feed them healthier meals at home. Today, the Department of Agriculture, Food, Nutrition and Consumer Services spends approximately $700 million annually on childhood nutrition education. They focus on small children developing better eating and fitness habits rather than weight loss. With proper nutrition and exercise, height and weight should balance out as they grow. If we want kids to eat healthier foods, we have to invest money into school nutrition programs so school lunches are healthier. If we want people to be more physically active, then there has to be safe places for them to exercise.

Although, most experts agree government funding will better target schools, parents have the greatest influence over what their children will eat. Normally, when families wise up and figure out what needs to happen, their children start to slim down. Parents care a lot about their children, and with proper education and the right tools, they really will try to do better. We have to demand that our schools and the principals who oversee them seek out the best sources of nutrition for our children. As I conclude this chapter, I want to leave you with a few tips and a couple of strategies that, if followed, will have your child in shape in no time. I want to help educate you and motivate you into taking action today, because, according to statistics, your child will have a 5-10 year shorter life span than you if you don't at least try.

In reality, these healthy habits should start at birth. However, it's still not too late. Children become overweight when there's an imbalance between their eating habits and physical activity. Therefore, it's best to incorporate changes in their daily regimen gradually. There are effective tactics for making even the pickiest eaters switch to healthier habits. One place to start is with your child's breakfast foods, as a vast majority of them are loaded with all types of sweeteners. First, if you can't pronounce all the ingredients and there are more than five ingredients listed on the package, your child shouldn't be eating that particular brand of cereal. Make plain water 90% of their primary source of hydration and give them soda and other sweetened beverages only before exercising.

Never allow them to drink any type of sweetened drink with their meals, again just water if they must have something. Try to incorporate more high water-content foods and minimize fried foods. These are just a few tactics you can start implementing today, and I've listed several more at the end of this chapter. Again, poverty is no excuse for obesity, and really no excuse for not living healthier and practicing healthy lifestyle habits. For example baking foods more often instead of frying is another great place to start. Water is a lot cheaper than soda or fruit juices. Oatmeal costs a lot less than most major brand cereals, and a bag of organic apples costs the same as a bag of Doritos chips.

If your neighborhood is not safe, children can do aerobic and callisthenic exercises in their bedrooms. You can easily put on a CD and walk, shadow box, jog, kick-box, do jumping jacks or dance in place. Children can also play fitness-oriented video games such as WiiFit/WiiActive or Kinex games. The key is to keep physically active even if it's only for 15 minutes per day or every other day. Whatever you do, don't settle for a sedentary lifestyle because it only leads to obesity and chronic degenerative diseases. Below is a list of tactics for getting your kids to eat healthier:

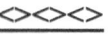

1. Switch out sugary cereals for low-sugar, fiber-rich organic cereals.

2. Give your kids bottled water for lunch and limit all sweetened beverages to just one per day, split into two servings if possible.

3. Switch to baked potato chips, and keep apples and nuts around the house for snacking.

4. Leave fruit out on the kitchen table or counter top.

5. Let your child have desserts, but never with a meal; always wait at least 2 hours after meals before serving dessert and serve with a glass of water.

6. Slip vegetables into their meat dishes and serve pasta with chunky organic tomato sauce.

7. Mix organic whole grain pancake or waffle mix batter with apples, applesauce or other fruits, except bananas and raisins, which are high-glycemic fruits that can cause a spike in blood sugar levels.

8. Serve a vegetable with lunch and dinner.

9. When eating fast food, skip the combo meals, and have a salad and water with your choice of meat or starch. When eating fast food, avoid combining high-fat protein with a high-glycemic starches.

10. Keep conversations positive; don't talk about losing weight, but improving healthier habits instead.

11. Buy organic dairy products and avoid non-organic dairy foods.

ROUTINE EXERCISE AND WEIGHT MANAGEMENT

CHAPTER IX

*J*ust imagine for a moment if one morning you happened to awaken and found that, overnight, you had managed to lose an astonishing 100 pounds. In amazement and utter exuberance, you quickly hopped out of bed and started frantically searching between the mattress, beneath the bed, behind the closet doors, maybe even among the clothes you tossed into the hamper before getting into bed the night before, desperately trying to find the fat that mysteriously disappeared so you can show it to all of your family members, friends, and coworkers.

Baffled and perplexed by what just happened, you sit on the edge of the bed and say to yourself, "Surely the diet pill I took before going to bed last night could not have worked that fast!" Next, you hear the alarm clock sound and you awaken, only to realize it was just a dream. Hesitantly, you ease out of bed to examine yourself in front of the mirror only to sadly discover the 100 pounds of fat is still stuck to your body.

So you decide to quickly hop back into bed and try to continue the dream where it left off. Sadly, millions of dieters live in dreamland, thinking they can continue eating as much as they want and still lose weight. Even the makers of the first diet weight loss pill approved by the FDA stress that no diet pill on the market can have this kind of impact on weight loss. They also stress that any diet plan must be combined with proper nutrition and exercise, two key behavior modification techniques I repeatedly emphasize in this book.

There are many weight loss and diet pill products out there that brag about being able to help you lose weight without exercising or getting sweaty. While all of these claims sound wonderful and exciting, they are not a healthy or a practical solution to permanent weight loss success. According to experts, exercise is vitally important to any successful weight loss program. Not only is exercise good for you, it accomplishes what no other diet pill in the world can do; it actually helps the body to naturally heal itself and reverse diseases like diabetes, heart disease, hypertension, depression, and yes, even obesity.

Medical experts say moderate exercise can help prevent the onset of many chronic degenerative diseases as well. It has been scientifically proven that people who exercise regularly actually live longer and healthier lives than those who don't. They also pay lower monthly medical costs for such things as prescription medications and doctor visits, and suffer from fewer annual illnesses. Exercise slows down the progression of aging and helps you look and feel younger. Medically, the veins and arteries of elderly people who exercise regularly are just as healthy as those of a young 20-year-old adult.

It was recently discovered that people with heart failure could benefit from exercise because it naturally enables the body to grow new veins and arteries, redirecting blood flow to the heart. With the body naturally healing itself in this manner, it further reduces the need for numerous heart stint operations doctors would otherwise have to perform. As I mentioned earlier, exercise makes the body more sensitive to insulin and quickly burns off excess glucose circulating in the blood, which helps to reverse Type 2 diabetes. Lower amounts of insulin have also been associated with a slower progression of aging.

But if all of these reasons weren't enough, I suppose one of the greatest benefits of exercise is the fact that it's the most effective way to cleanse the blood of toxins, cellular waste, and accumulated debris. It also allows the body to burn excess calories and fatty acids, while at the same time building lean muscle mass. When you build lean muscle mass, gaining weight becomes more difficult because lean muscle keeps your metabolism elevated, burning extra calories even when your body is at rest.

I'm quite sure many of you are familiar with community neighborhood watch groups that are spread throughout the United States. This is where neighbors come together and agree to watch each other's property by vigilantly protecting and guarding against theft and vandalism. Any suspicious activity in the neighborhood is then immediately reported to the local authorities. From the term neighborhood watch, I coined my own phrase: "neighborhood walk." A neighborhood walk involves neighbors coming together with other residents of that particular community and walking for up to 30 minutes several times per week. Residents meet at pre-designated areas such as local parks, schools, or right in the community, and exercise together. Since this is a cooperative community effort, as many people in the neighborhood as possible, from little toddlers and their parents, to the eldest senior citizens, are a part of the effort, encouraged and if necessary escorted to the staging areas where everyone stretches and hydrates properly before exercising. Can you imagine? Instead of watching out for burglars, neighbors could actually monitor each other's waistlines, as excessive weight can blindly rob your neighbors of their health and wealth.

I recommend appointing a Team Captain who assigns several Sergeants-at-Arms who are responsible for the coordination and overall safety of these short community walks. These leaders should be certified in CPR and carry a small first aid kit and a cell phone. You could even bring along the family pet, and in inclement weather arrange to use the gymnasium at your local school or religious center. A positive byproduct of this program would be safer and friendlier neighborhoods, resulting in lower crime rates, as people get to know each other better and show a genuine concern for each other's health. Listen, my friend; walking is free! It costs you absolutely nothing, so you really have no excuse for not taking advantage of this incredible opportunity to better the lives of yourself and other people.

Humans were not created to sit around immobile for an extended period of time. In the past 100 to 150 years, the majority of the population has become immobilized. Today, between commuting back and forth to work, playing video games, watching TV, and sitting behind a desk at work, the average person gets very little physical activity. This sedentary lifestyle and physical inactivity is just as hazardous to your health as practicing unhealthy eating habits.

According to medical experts, moderate smokers who exercise regularly are reported to be healthier than non-smokers who don't exercise at all. The same is true for people with high blood pressure. Even if you are not overweight, exercise should be a part of your normal routine because it greatly enhances optimum health.

Moderate exercise regularly reduces body fat, increases lean muscle mass, lowers blood pressure, lowers insulin resistance, and raises HDL while lowering LDL cholesterol levels, having a positive effect on the entire body. By now, it should not surprise you to hear that millions of Americans suffer from illnesses that can be prevented or improved through regular physical activity.

Our young people today can barely run three miles without passing out or stopping every few yards to catch their breath. We accept this as routine because we're out of shape and don't exercise ourselves. Listen, I don't care if it's just 15 minutes; turn off the TV, put the game controller down, and get up and exercise! If you're too tired to work out after work, then go to bed 15 minutes earlier and wake up 15 minutes earlier to exercise. I can't overstress the importance of making exercise a lifestyle habit; it really is a matter of life and death.

Your physical well-being is just as important as your job, family, friends, religion, and any other things in your life. With all the advantages we have today like transportation, refrigeration, and health clubs, you would expect that we would be a healthier nation. Actually, we would be healthier if it were not for two underlying issues I keep emphasizing: lack of exercise and poor dietary habits. Years ago I was told by friends, who were concerned for my health, that I should stop jogging so much. They were afraid I would damage my knees from the constant pounding on the concrete pavement. I was warned that by the time I turned 30, my knees would be totally shot and I wouldn't be able to run at all.

Well, all I can say is I thank God I didn't follow their advice and stop jogging. Today I still jog quite a bit and sometimes I'll run up to 20 miles per week if I have the time. What's amazing is the fact that my knees (and for that matter my entire body) has never felt better. I actually look forward to running more than I do to sitting down for a meal. When my 6-year-old daughter was younger, I use to push her along in her stroller as I ran on our scenic tour of rolling hills and lush green pastures. Today, we go for long brisk walks, which she really enjoys and looks forward to. I am trying to instill in her the values and benefits that exercise can offer while she is still young. By doing this she will grow up viewing exercise as just a routine part of everyday life and not some boring chore.

Running has become therapeutic for me, sort of like an outlet from all of the stresses and hassles of everyday life. It is my personal belief that the lifestyle changes I implemented earlier in my life have made a major positive impact on my health today. If you think you're too old or over-the-hill, guess what; you're not! An increasing number of studies continue to show that it's never too late to start exercising; even small improvements in physical fitness can significantly lower the risk of developing certain diseases associated with obesity and premature death.

If you're out of shape and a couch potato, don't expect to go out and run in the Marine Corps Marathon. Begin with 15 to 20 minutes of light exercise or a brisk daily walk, and then gradually increase the intensity and duration of how long you work out. Even after age 50, exercise can add health and active years to one's life. Elderly people can prolong their lives and lessen their dependency on costly medications by simply walking regularly. They can even reduce loss of muscle mass through resistance training. Bone density, muscle mass, and strength can be maintained or even enhanced through exercise because these organs only respond to resistance training. Stiffness and loss of balance that accompanies aging can be greatly reduced by simply incorporating flexibility exercises.

It is amazing the number of people who don't exercise, yet expect to miraculously maintain optimum health. Walking is one of the easiest and most beneficial exercises one can do. If you have children it can be a lot of fun because they love being outdoors, and they also love spending time with their parents!

Certain types of cancers, clogged arteries, hypertension, and osteoporosis, all associated with obesity, have been prevented or greatly marginalized with routine exercise. Numerous studies have shown that exercise training in coronary artery disease patients improves survival. You can also reverse and greatly marginalize Type 2 diabetes by losing just 7-10% of your total body weight, making routine exercise a part of your daily life, and incorporating a few healthy dietary habits. As more and more cultures around the world adopt western dietary habits, Type 2 diabetes in particular, as well as hypertension and obesity, are starting to reach epidemic proportions. People who engage in regular exercise, like walking briskly, can lower their risk for diabetes without losing a pound. If you are taking insulin or suffering from diabetes, however, take special precautions (discussed below) before embarking on a workout program.

Nerve damage from diabetes is horrific, causing blindness and loss of hearing; it is a leading cause of kidney failure and prevents healing when injuries occur. Blood sugar normally rises to 170 from a fasting level of 110 after you eat a meal. When levels reach 170, the pancreas releases large amounts of insulin which causes blood sugars to gradually fall. Diabetics either don't produce enough insulin or cannot respond adequately to this rise in blood sugar levels, so their blood sugar levels rise above 170 and stay elevated. Under normal conditions, glucose is harmless, but when your blood sugars remain too high, glucose begins to stick to your cells. Once it is attached to a cell, sugar cannot be removed and is converted into sorbitol, an alcohol sugar created by an enzyme called aldose reductase. Sorbitol can eventually destroy cells and cause damaged arteries, increasing the risk of heart attack.

For some reason this process is elevated in diabetics and causes dangerous complications over time. Sorbitol can't exit quickly from cells and is not used by the body, so it accumulates and attracts water. This causes cells to enlarge, resulting in the development of cataracts as well as nerve, eye, and kidney damage. However, through regular exercise, the liver and muscles removes excess glucose from the blood, which helps regulate insulin levels after a meal—but that's only if they are emptied to begin with. Watching your sugar intake, but more importantly exercising, can keep sugar levels in check, preventing nerve cell damage and enabling the body to heal itself. The following precautions should be taken before starting an exercise program, especially if you are a diabetic:

Do not exercise if your blood sugar is above 350. Make sure you eat first, take medications, and keep bread, potato chips, or honey around in case your blood sugar levels drop too low during exercise. You may even want to consult with a personal trainer to make sure you get the proper amount of exercise. An exercise program should start slowly and build up to more strenuous activities. One of the greatest benefits of being physically active is the reduced risk of heart attack and death. For an overweight person, exercise is vitally important, as it is for anyone who has diabetes or other risk factors related to heart disease.

The Harvard Alumni study found that increased physical activity from 500 calories to 2,000 calories per week showed a reduction in death from heart attacks. Other studies from the Lipid Research Clinics found that men who were physically fit were less likely to die from heart attacks than men who were out of shape. Exercise shouldn't be used solely to lose weight, but to change the condition of the body and make it healthier. People who exercise are more likely to maintain the weight they lose, as opposed to those who don't exercise.

In addition to increased energy levels, exercise increases nervous system activity and also feelings of well-being. If you exercise, you have a lower risk of depression because of weight gain. Exercise helps maintain full functioning and independence among the elderly. Physical activity reduces oxygen demand, the tendency for blood clots to form in arteries that have narrowed, and increases elasticity in the arteries. Women who suffer from difficult menstrual cycles can benefit greatly from routine exercise. However, don't expect any overnight miracles, as the benefits of exercise occur gradually and become evident over a one or two month period.

Also, exercise releases large amounts of the hormone dopamine into the bloodstream. With this hormone present, the feeling of hunger greatly diminishes. This is an excellent way to manage your weight without starving yourself. It is also the healthiest approach to use, because it will actually strengthen and heal the body both inside and out. This is something dieting, diet pills, and gastric bypass surgery will never be able to totally accomplish. You could take over 100 different types of medications and spend thousands of dollars every week and still wouldn't get the same benefits that regular exercise can produce. Routine exercise accomplishes all of this, keeps you from becoming overweight, and doesn't cost you a dime. So what is your excuse? You can increase your personal net-worth and improve your quality of life all at the same time.

The chart on page 95 shows the calories burned during certain types of exercises. This is not a complete list of all physical activities, but it will give you a little insight into what types of exercises you may want to do. The calorie information listed in the chart is based on one hour of physical activity covering three separate weight classes. The numbers given may fluctuate up or down and are provided strictly for educational purposes. If you are suffering from medical conditions, it is advised you consult with your physician before implementing any of the exercises listed below.

When you do exercise, make sure you get plenty of potassium daily to help prevent muscle spasms and cramping. Celery, prunes, squash, oranges, and drinking organic grape and prune juices are all excellent sources of potassium.

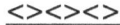

Activity	Calories burned per weight (per 1 hour of exercise)		
	135 lbs	150 lbs	195 lbs
Aerobics general	350	418	500
Aerobics high impact	418	485	609
Aerobics low impact	270	380	440
Basketball game	480	580	685
Bicycling leisure	246	286	351
Bicycling moderate	496	585	698
Bicycling vigorously	595	746	875
Bicycle stationary 1	189	224	250
Bicycle stationary 2	290	360	440
Bicycle stationary 3	413	493	604
Bicycle stationary 4	635	745	916
Boxing punching bag	365	430	535
Boxing sparring	540	645	786
Canoeing rowing	177	211	259
Dancing fast	354	422	518
Dancing slow	170	201	245
Dancing general	266	317	358
Football touch	476	536	690
Football competitive	531	633	776
Golf general	236	281	355
Golf miniature	177	220	259
Jogging	413	419	604
Rope jumping	710	850	1040
Running	628	833	1035
Running track	595	714	870
Roller skating	420	495	610
Skiing	420	500	615
Soccer	450	620	840
Softball	300	360	440
Swimming laps	550	650	750
Swimming leisurely	385	428	535
Tennis	416	497	609
Volleyball	475	568	595
Walking	425	493	615
Walking track	294	365	434
Water aerobics	240	285	314
Weight lifting	215	235	410

20 Minute Exercise Program

The following exercises should be completed within 20 minutes. Take 15-second breaks between each exercise. These exercises should be performed 3 to 4 times a week or more if you desire. Try to do at least 3 to 4 sets of exercises within 20 minutes. The exercises are designed to help develop lean muscle mass as they work on every muscle group in the body. Lean muscle mass allows you to burn calories and fat even while your body is at rest. Instead of losing pounds, you will lose inches, developing a much more contoured and shapely body.

Jumping Jacks

If you are unable to do regular jumping jacks because of knee or joint problems, simply go through the motions without allowing your feet to leave the floor: slightly bend the knees and wave your arms as if you are doing jumping jacks. Perform 100 jumping jacks in 2 minute to complete one set.

Push-Ups

Perform 20 push-ups in one minute. If you are unable to do regular push-ups, simply place your hands under your shoulders and raise the body by pushing down on the palms but keep your knees on the floor. Be sure to push up using just your arms and upper body. Do 20 push-ups to complete one set.

Cross Crunch Sit-Ups

Lay flat on your back and cross your right knee over your left knee. Pull your left elbow up toward your right knee. Repeat this back and forth side-ways motion 20 times and then switch knees and do 20 reps on the other side. Perform both positions in 1 minute to complete one set.

Bend and Reach

Stand with your hands resting on your hips and your feet shoulder-width apart. In one complete motion bend over and touch your toes, come up and touch your hips, continue upward extending your arms and hands far above your head, then bring your hands back down to your hips. This is one complete rep. Do 10reps in 30 seconds to complete one set.

Weighted Squats

Standing with feet just beyond shoulder-width, bring your 20-40 pound dumbbell weights up to your chest and hold them there. Now squat down and push yourself back up. Perform 8 squats to complete one set.

Curls and Overhead Extensions

Stand with feet shoulder-width apart, holding 20-40 pound dumbbells down to your side with palms facing forward. Bring right dumb-bell up to your shoulder in a curling motion. Once at your shoulder, rotate your arm so that the palm is facing forward, extend your right hand with dumb-bell above your head while simultaneously bringing left dumb-bell up to your shoulder and rotating your palm forward.

As you begin to lower the right dumb-bell, start raising the left dumb-bell above your head. While lowering the left dumb-bell, bring the right dumb-bell back down to your side, returning it to the original starting position. Continue lowering left dumb-bell, returning it to your left side. This is one complete rep. Repeat these steps 8 times to complete one set.

LOSING WEIGHT PERMANENTLY
BREAKING BAD HABITS

CHATER X

I am sure many of you are quite familiar with the old cliché, "birds of a feather flock together." Believe it or not, as it relates to gaining weight and obesity, there is a lot of truth to this statement. Scientists recently discovered that obese people with obese family and friends tend to socialize together more than their counterparts of normal weight. In fact, they found such a strong connection between obese people and those with whom they were most likely to associate, calling this a "social contagion." Dr. Nicholas Christakis, a professor of medical sociology at Harvard Medical School and coauthor of a report featured in the New England Journal of Medicine, asserted their findings showing that obesity is contagious—in a social sense, of course, so don't panic.

I'm sure you can vividly remember family gatherings of your own, with everyone sitting around and gorging themselves while socializing. In fact, when people eat together in groups, calorie counting seems to go right out the window fairly quickly. It's easy to eat a few extra servings while you are talking, laughing, and having fun. The aforementioned researchers discovered that people whose siblings become obese were themselves 40% more likely to grow obese. In fact, the study further illustrated if someone became obese, their friends were 57% more likely to become obese over time.

The researchers used their report as the first conclusive study to show how obesity spreads from person to person through social networks. On that note, perhaps if everyone got together and participated in healthier behavior modification techniques, just the opposite would occur. Married couples were 37% more likely to become obese if one of the spouses were to become obese. I actually had a chance to personally witness this phenomenon. On one occasion, some friends and I visited one of America's favorite all-you-can-eat buffet restaurants. (By the way, all-you-can-eat buffets

99

are almost unheard of in parts of the world outside of the U.S.) I deliberately decided not to eat any of the foods at the buffet, and instead sipped on a glass of lemon-water while observing the people dinning around us.

In the room adjacent to ours, there was an unusually large group of about 30 or so people seated at a table, ranging in ages from little toddlers to senior citizens. It was quite clear that many of them were family members, or related in some way or another. Because they all sat together at one long table it was very easy to observe their eating habits. What shocked me most was the fact that more than two-thirds of the people at the table were grossly overweight, and about half of them were obese. As I sat and watched them happily converse and laugh together, I also thought to myself how they were slowly and insidiously destroying their health and endangering their lives.

It was as if they were all on auto pilot, repeatedly visiting the entree bars and loading their plates to full capacity. In fact, it appeared as though the amount of food on their plates was proportionate to the enormous size of their bodies. I noted that as they gorged themselves, they were totally oblivious to what was going on around them. When dessert time came, it was the same thing repeated again: over-indulgence. When they got up to leave the restaurant, almost half of them could barely walk. You could see their physical discomfort as many struggled to their feet and hobbled for the exit doors. Even more distressing was watching the little toddlers who were just as obese as the adults and appeared physically hampered by their weight as well.

As I watched, I became disheartened, imagining these poor helpless little children who more than likely wouldn't outlive their parents, because children are at a much higher risk of dying prematurely from diseases associated with obesity than obese adults. This incident clearly supports the findings of the researchers who reported that if someone's friends become obese, that person's chances of becoming obese increases by more than half. These findings hold true for people who live great distances apart as well. If the group I observed that day in the restaurant was having a family reunion, then it further proves obesity is not just an individual problem but a collective social problem.

This brings me to my next point; your friends and family members can be your worst enemy when you are trying to practice healthy lifestyle habits. I know this all too well. For years my family has tried to get me to revert back to my old unhealthy eating habits. I was always the brunt of cynical food jokes at family gatherings, and was made fun of quite a bit. In fact, some of my family and friends thought I had actually gone crazy because I declined to emulate their hazardous eating behavior. Don't worry, I never took any of their jokes personally, I simply knew what I had to do if I was going to avoid becoming another tragic statistic. It is amazing how life has a way of reversing itself, because today most of my family members and friends seek my advice regarding their health issues as they struggle with their own weight-related diseases.

I saw first-hand what kind of long-term damage unhealthy eating habits can cause. At the age of 13, I witnessed my father suffer a massive debilitating stroke that left him paralyzed and vocally impaired for the rest of his life. I'll never forget the loud hard thumping sound I heard coming from my parents' bedroom as my father fell to the floor. When I ran into the room to see what had happened, I saw my father lying helplessly paralyzed on the floor, totally disoriented and unable to speak or move his body. Just moments earlier, my dad had awakened me to have breakfast with him, as he did each morning before heading off to work. But from that day on he would never again awaken me to have breakfast with him. In just a matter of seconds, a man whom I had always seen as tough as nails and as strong as an ox, had been transformed into a speechless paralytic.

After the doctors conducted their tests, they told us my father should have never survived his ordeal, and it was a miracle he was still alive. It turned out my dad was as tough as nails after all, and he was determined not to allow his own children to grow up fatherless as he had. Sometime later, it was determined the hypertension that caused my father's stroke was a hereditary condition, and we were all at a greater risk of suffering from a stroke. I made a decision from that day onward that I would not allow food to be my enemy and destroy my health. I vowed to learn how to incorporate healthy behavior modification techniques that would help make food friendly to me and preserve my health. It took some time for me to evolve and fully grasp the concepts I live by today, but I was determined not to give up on myself.

Hypertension, also known as a silent killer, is the third leading cause of death in this country. It is directly tied to excessive weight, unhealthy eating habits, smoking, and a sedentary lifestyle. Over the years I have been adamant about not allowing relatives or friends to persuade me into altering my eating habits to mimic theirs. If you're going to have success in any weight loss program, you must have the same tenacity and not give into peer pressure. Look at it this way, if one of your best friends was about to rob a bank and requested your assistance, the average person would decline such a request without thinking twice about it. You'll have to have this same type of mind-set when avoiding unhealthy eating habits, as they will eventually rob you of your health.

For the most part, we like to spend time with people who are similar to us, because they make us feel comfortable. In fact, researchers report we tend to eat for longer periods of time when we are with friends. Most of us try to use good table manners by not leaving the table until everyone has finished eating. In many ways, eating is almost like going shopping, in that the longer you shop the more money you end up spending. The more time you spend at a table with family and friends, the more food you tend to eat, according to psychologists who say this trend is almost mathematically predictable. They report if you eat with another person, you will, on average, consume up to 35% more food than if you eat alone.

If you add six or more people to your party, this percentage rises as high as 96%. If you cut this number down to just four people, they say you will likely eat about 75% more calories than if you were to eat alone. Oftentimes, you will come across entire families where every member is overweight, as close friends and family members tend to weigh the same. It can seem almost impossible for a dieting person to lose weight in a family in which everyone is overweight, but it can be done if you model yourself after the right people.

By hanging around people who are conscious about their eating habits, and who practice healthier behavior modification techniques, you will inadvertently pick up their habits and not feel pressured into overeating. This will allow you to separate yourself from the millions of other people who resort to dieting, or who follow the latest dietary fad. In this country alone, Americans spent a staggering $50 billion on diet and weight-loss products in 2010, and the majority of them failed to lose weight permanently. Today, everywhere you look, people are either dieting or about to start on a new one.

In fact, it seems as if ever since I can remember, I've always known someone who was on some type of newly discovered diet, including myself at one time or another. It seems as though we're always desperately trying to lose weight. Many people dread gaining weight as much as they fear being diagnosed with cancer. People so fear this, they remain nervously preoccupied with the dreadful idea of it happening to them. Sadly, of all the people who spent $50 billion to lose weight last year, more than two thirds wasted their hard-earned money, because according to government studies, 65% of all dieters regain their weight back within 1 year. Further studies concluded, over a 5-year period, 97% of all dieters regain the weight they lost, and even end up weighing more than they did before they started dieting.

Let us stop here for a second and do the math: $50 billion spent on people trying to lose weight, multiplied by 5 years = $250 billion.

Why are so many people resorting to diets in this country when the overwhelming proof is that they don't really work? Why do so many people go through all of the trouble to lose weight, only to watch as they gain it all back plus a few extra pounds? Why do so many people continually spend billions of their hard earned dollars, only to end up throwing it all away? Why do so many people devote so much of their precious time, effort, and energy, only to accomplish dismal results? I don't care how you slice it or dice it, 97% is a complete failure. If you were hoping to graduate from college but failed to pass 97% of the required curriculum well, you get my point.

The fact is diet pills, video tapes, CDs, diet books, prepackaged meals, weight loss centers, and medical interventions are simply not the real solution to long-term permanent weight loss. These approaches are ineffective at dealing with the little person inside of you—you know, the real you that no one really knows about. This person stares back at you every time you look in the mirror. This person discusses your weight problems with you, and is there when you make promises again and again about how you're going to make major changes. This person is just as inescapable as your own shadow, following you wherever you go. There is nothing you can do to get rid of this little person.

This person inside you says, "I really don't want to be overweight and obese, will you please help me?" This is you who crying out when no one else is around, because you are tired of fighting the bulge, and wish there was an easier way out. This you when you're all alone and hidden behind closed doors, when you retire that diet for just one night so you can go and pig out. This is the real you, the one that cannot be helped with diet pills, video tapes, CDs, diet books, prepackaged meals, weight loss centers, or gastric bypass surgery. These things cannot change the underlying issues and conditions that are causing you to gain weight.

A close friend of mine once told me about his cousin who had her stomach stapled in order to lose weight and help stop her from overeating. On one occasion she became gravely ill because she had overeaten one too many times, causing the staples in her stomach to rip apart. Her medical approach to dieting had failed bringing her dangerously close to death's door. This all happened because she hadn't incorporated better behavior modification techniques in order to make permanent lifestyle changes. She took the shortcut by way of medical intervention, which inadvertently led to her bleeding internally and developing a dangerous infection. She had temporarily succeeded in transforming her body, but her mind was where the battle truly needed to be won.

I'm quite certain that at some point she could feel the need to push away the plate, but decided to satisfy her eating compulsions instead. The fact that her stomach had been stapled was proof that at some point she'd had a conscious discussion with her inner self. The next step, however, should have been for her to implement healthier behavior modification techniques. This is where the true approach to long-term permanent weight loss begins. In fact, people shouldn't be on diets anyway, because weight management occurs naturally as a result of healthier lifestyle habits, which also prevents unwanted weight gain. If more people incorporated healthier behavior modification techniques instead of dieting, weight loss would be

97% successful instead of the dismal failure repeatedly seen year after year.

Listen; I too was once trapped, going on diet after diet, always battling with myself, trying to keep off those extra pounds, and constantly seeking out the next new diet plan because the last five had failed. It wasn't until I decided to stop dieting and start incorporating behavior modification techniques that I actually lost the weight and was able to keep it off permanently. Once I stopped the dieting cycle and made behavior modification a part of my daily lifestyle, the weight just naturally dropped off effortlessly. Now, the greatest benefits I experienced were not the pounds I was able to shed, but the internal healing that took place. Instead of changing dietary habits and principles just to lose weight, it should become your lifestyle every moment of the day to improve the overall condition of your health.

A lot of people are fit but not healthy, and that's the reason lifestyle changes are far more important than just losing weight. There are many factors that contribute to weight gain, but there are only two real reasons why people continue to gain weight at such an accelerated rate: The unlimited availability and access to a myriad of different foods 24 hours a day, and the unhealthy lifestyle choices people habitually practice.

Obesity expert Dr. Xavier Pisunyer of Columbia University in New York says people with excess fat tend to have higher free fatty acids circulating in their blood. There has been some data to suggest that higher circulating free fatty acids could be a risk factor for increased cardiac arrhythmia. Earlier in the book, I briefly mentioned the half-ton man who came very close to dying because of his weight. He had struggled with weight problems since kindergarten, when he weighed 90 pounds. By the time he reached middle school his weight had ballooned to 250 pounds. He most likely inherited bad eating habits passed down from his father and grandfather, who both weighed more than 300 pounds each. This is definitely a good example of obesity being a social disease.

As an adult, this man worked as a chef and had access to food whenever he wanted it. This choice was to his detriment because he hadn't learned behavior modification techniques that would have prevented him from ever becoming morbidly obese. He finally realized if he was going to save his life, he had to drastically change his behavior about food and become physically active. By the way, had he applied this approach initially, medical intervention would have never been necessary. He is not alone, as over 100,000 people are morbidly obese in this country and they are the fastest growing segment of the population. With all the new diet products, self-help books, weight loss centers, and advances in surgical procedures available today, people are still continuing to pack on the pounds. Some have even been misguided into believing they suffer from some type of medical disorder that causes them to spontaneously gain an extra 150-200 pounds.

Researchers have conclusively proven this not the case. They stress that this epidemic is strictly a behavioral problem, and not a medical or scientific condition. In other words, the obesity epidemic has nothing to do with medicine or science, but unhealthy nutritional habits that people habitually choose to practice. So many people are suffering with debilitating medical conditions that are directly related to obesity. So many children are swollen and uncomfortable-looking as they struggle to lug around all that excess weight. You can't go shopping without seeing people driving themselves around in mobile carts because obesity prevents them from being able to walk.

Before bank debit cards and ATM machines became widely available, people had access to money only during normal banking hours. Consequently, they spent less and saved more. Today, with 24 hour ATM machines, people have unlimited access to money, so they spend a whole lot more and save a lot less. Look at the invisible link between increased credit and debit card usage and the explosion of overweight people. Unlimited access equals more use and abuse. Either way, it appears as though having more may not always be the best option for many people.

Researchers at Cornell University and Penn State University have repeatedly demonstrated that people tend to eat more when served larger portions. Researchers further noted that eating slowly helps us to better savor our food, creating more satisfaction even with smaller portions. Now, I know you can't force the restaurants and convenience stores in your neighborhood to stop operating 24 hours a day in order for you not to have access to food wherever and whenever you want it, but you can use behavior modification techniques and not allow that food to have access to you.

The food we eat today is specifically produced to make us want and crave more of it, even if it is totally unhealthy. For example, everybody knows too much sugar isn't good for your health. You've heard it ever since you were a little toddler from your parents and grandparents. The food industry knows that sugar is bad for you as well, but it also knows without sugar, many customers won't buy their products. Without customers, there is really no reason to be in business. For this reason, almost everything you buy is loaded with sugar, and just because the word "sugar" is not listed in the ingredients doesn't mean it doesn't contain sugar. There are all kinds of chemical derivative sweeteners like high fructose corn syrup, potassium sorbate, sodium erthrobate, saccharin, aspartame, Splenda, neotame, acesulfame, sucralose, sucrose, maltose, maltodextrin, dextrose, sorbitol, corn syrup, barley malt, and caramel, just to name a few.

All these sugars are health hazards to the human body because most of them are chemical derivatives, and they are consumed in very large quantities. The key is balancing your diet with more fresh fruits, vegetables and water. This is exactly the type of diet our grandparents ate years before the current obesity epidemic came about. Today, in many countries where commercially-processed foods have replaced traditional diets of fresh fruits, vegetables, and lean meats, people are experiencing a dramatic increase in obesity rates and obesity-related diseases. The recommended consumption of sugar by the USDA is an average of no more than 10 teaspoons a day for a healthy adult, which, in my opinion, is still too much,

Most of our toddlers and young children surpass the USDA daily recommendation of sugar consumption by the time they finish breakfast. These chemical sweeteners are just empty calories that take the place of real nutrients. While we eat and pack on the pounds, we are really starving ourselves. Food is plentiful, but the average diet is very low in nutrition, according to many experts. For example, Britain is also suffering with its own obesity tragedy, and although it is apparent that many British people are overweight, it is estimated nearly 2 million are also most likely malnourished. Experts note the poor state of the average British diet is high in unhealthy fats, carbohydrates, salt, and calories, rendering it nutritionally void. Even though food is plentiful in Great Britain, such a diet leaves its consumers malnourished.

People may be consuming too much food however a vast majority do not eat enough fresh fruits and vegetables. There is a widely held misconception that if you're overweight, you must be well-nourished. According to some experts, the food rationing system during World War II offered Britons more nutrition than what they're eating today. While many overweight and obese people are not in any immediate danger of starvation, other obesity-related complications are possible, such as diabetes, hypertension, and heart disease. The national diet in Britain is so hazardous, the United Kingdom's Food Standard Agency recommended folic acid added to the nation's flour—a lack of this essential vitamin in pregnant women has been linked to birth defects.

The main source of the problem again goes back to the rise in consumption of processed foods and fast foods. Our entire digestive process is thrown completely off-kilter by these foods, and uncontrollable weight gain kicks in as insulin levels remain abnormally elevated, constantly forcing fat into fat cells. As these fat cells reach their stretching capacity, signals are sent to the surrounding tissue, triggering the production of new fat cells. People grow fatter and fatter, with some actually becoming horrifically engorged in fat.

I want to take a moment to talk about Chinese food, as it is very popular worldwide. Most of the foods in these restaurants are loaded with unhealthy fat, sodium, and calories. For example, a single serving of General Tso's chicken has almost 3,200 milligrams of sodium, 1,300 calories and 11 grams of saturated fat. That's before you include the rice and egg rolls, adding another 400 calories and 400 milligrams of sodium. However, the average person doesn't stop there; he or she also drinks some sort of soft drink, instead of drinking lots of water to immediately neutralize and flush this meal out of his or her body.

I want to point out here that the traditional Chinese diet tastes nothing like what is being served in your local fast-food restaurants. The traditional Chinese diet consists mainly of steamed rice, sautéed or steamed fresh vegetables, and lean meats like poultry and fish, all of which are almost entirely void of heavy sauces. The drink of choice is hot tea, desserts are never served with the main meal, and foods are rarely deep-fried. If you ate like this, you would never have a problem with your weight. American Chinese food is bad for your waistline and blood pressure, and the large amounts of sodium can contribute to hypertension, especially in sodium-sensitive people.

Mexican and Italian food are just as unhealthy, because they are loaded with high amounts of saturated fat, which has been implicated in causing heart disease. People should consider single meals served at these restaurants as two separate dishes and not one. Because portion sizes are so large, half of these meals can be taken home and eaten for lunch the next day. Avoid the heavy sauces at all costs, or if at all possible, make your own. In the end, it's up to you, the consumer, to request the healthier choices from the menu. And don't be fooled by the vegetable choices, as they score just as poorly in the amounts of sodium and carbohydrates. A plate of stir-fried greens, for example, has about 900 calories and 2,200 milligrams of sodium. The rest of this chapter will deal with what you will need in order to lose weight permanently and improve your overall health. You are guaranteed to shed the pounds and keep them off by modifying your behavior using the rest of the information provided in this chapter. Remember, you were not born overweight or obese; these conditions manifested over a period of time.

The first step to losing weight permanently is to start with an understanding of the psychology of food. Many people live to eat instead of eating to live. They have grown up with traditional eating habits that have been passed down to them for generations. The traditional meal consists of meat, potatoes or other starches, various types of breads, dessert, and a sugary ice cold drink with almost every meal except breakfast, which is usually some type of highly processed concoction. By the end of the day you've consumed enough sugar to fill a coffee cup, with most of these sugars in the form of some kind of synthetically altered substance that can adversely impact the liver. You bypass fresh fruits and vegetables because they just aren't as appealing to your palate as junk food. If you want to really lose weight and keep it off, the following behavior modification techniques will get you started in the right direction:

First, you must change your mentality about what constitutes a real complete meal. Second, you must disregard the notion that you need three large meals a day. Third, you must educate yourself in proper nutrition, hydration, and physical activity. Mastering these three key strategic areas of health are fundamentally paramount to permanent and successful weight loss.

A real meal doesn't have to include all the food groups listed on the USDA food pyramid. You can eat small meals encompassing a variety of different types of foods spread out over the course of the entire day. For example, I consider two apples or a cup of seeded grapes as constituting a meal. A half-cup of raw almonds or cashews could be another meal. A serving of baked chicken with two sides of vegetables is a complete meal. The side dishes should always be your choice of vegetables and a nice large green leafy salad without fattening salad dressing.

Also, poverty is no excuse for obesity, as poor people tend to have a lot of unhealthy nutritional habits that are probably caused by social and environmental factors. However, it is just as easy to boil or bake meats as it is to fry them, and boiling is a lot healthier than frying. Baked French fries are better for your health than fried ones any day of the week.

Water is good for flushing and cleansing the colon and every cell in the body. Amazingly, we use water to wash our clothes, cars, dishes, bodies, and pets. If water is so necessary for washing and cleansing, why don't we drink more of it? If it's good for all the external purposes we use it for, certainly it must be good for internal cleansing as well. Weight loss can be greatly optimized by drinking more water.

Some people try getting by on low-fat or fat-free diets, but as I stated before, the human body needs fat to function properly, so a fat-free diet is very unhealthy. It's not so much the fat itself, but the type of fat consumed. Low-fat dairy products are often loaded with sugar or artificial sweeteners, even though they may not appear on the label.

Exercise of any type, especially brisk walking, jogging, jumping rope, or swimming, is very beneficial for weight loss and overall wellness. It doesn't matter if you exercise for 20 minutes or an hour, two or more times per week, just as long as you exercise. Exercise will help oxygenate the body and keep the hormones dopamine and serotonin circulating in the blood, which will greatly help curb uncontrollable hunger urges. I like to do a workout routine

I've developed when I don't have time to get out and jog. I begin by doing jumping jacks for 5 minutes, followed by 100 sit-ups and 40 push-ups executed in three consecutive sets. I have designed an exercise plan outlined in chapter 9 that will greatly enhance your weight loss experience.

Now, of course, if you are just starting out, you want to go easy depending on your size and ability. I don't like using scales because they can complicate weight loss, as the body is transformed from fat into more lean muscle mass. Muscle weighs more than fat, so the scale may not move much. Instead of seeing a dramatic drop in weight, you may notice a leaner, toner, body. I personally allow my weight to fluctuate between 5-10 pounds in either direction of my normal body weight. I think this is healthy, because it keeps me from panicking and worrying about my weight, as excess worry and stress can also complicate weight management. In addition, 5 or 10 pounds for an active person eating whole grain foods and healthy fats is very easy to burn off. So I leave myself this little extra cushion, and so far, it has worked very effectively.

Listen, I am no different than any of you and grew up eating all the wrong types of foods and practicing unhealthy eating habits. If I can lose weight and keep it off, so can you. We are no different; healthy behavior modification techniques and consistency is all that it takes. This approach will work. I promise it will, as long as you do your part.

35 BEHAVIOR MODIFICATION TECHNIQUES

CHATER XI

*B*elow, I've listed 35 key behavior modification techniques for a successful weight loss career. These techniques are designed to help you manage your weight permanently, safely and effectively. Some medical conditions may have to be addressed first as they may hinder weight loss. These are the techniques I have incorporated for over 30 years; they have helped to make my weight loss career a successful one without dieting, diet pills, or medical intervention.

1. Proper Meal Combining, A: Always eat animal proteins (steak, chicken, pork, etc.) and cooked starches (rice, potatoes, pasta, etc.) separately. The exception to this rule is eating lean meats like baked, broiled or steamed fish. When eating animal protein, combine it with a large leafy green salad and two vegetable dishes of your choice. Don't worry about serving sizes or counting calories; as your stomach begins to shrink you will naturally start eating less. The key here is to not starve yourself or feel deprived. Make your own salad dressing (instructions for this will be in chapter 12), or buy an organic dressing.

2. Proper Meal Combining, B: When eating cooked starchy foods the same rules apply; skip the cooked meats and sugary drinks and have some vegetables and a large green salad. Don't worry about serving sizes or counting calories; as your stomach begins to shrink you will naturally start eating less.

3. Proper Meal Combining, C: Raw plant-based proteins (nuts, seeds, algae, ect.) and non-refined, non-dried, raw plant-based carbohydrates (apples, pears, peaches, ect.) make a great snack and are a good source of quick energy. The combination of fruits and nuts is very effective in suppressing hunger and food cravings. I recommend restricting the nut intake to small 1oz serving sizes.

4. Hydration: Drinking beverages with meals is not recommended, however, if you must drink something it should be just plain water (or hot tea (green), which naturally helps the body burn fat. All sweetened beverages should be consumed by themselves and never with a meal. It is best to drink sweetened beverages a half hour to an hour prior to exercising, as this will immediately remove excess sugar from circulation and make the body more sensitive to insulin.

This dual action helps to prevent the onset of diabetes, heart disease, and hypertension, while at the same time preventing fat storage, which leads to excessive weight gain. Sweetened beverages should be consumed sparingly, totally combined to no more than 10% of your total weekly hydration intake. You can take one 12-ounce serving of your favorite sweetened beverage and split it in half. This will give you two 6-ounce servings to be consumed between meals or before working out.

5. Dessert: You can have your cake and ice cream too, but just don't eat them with the main course. Desserts should be eaten preferably 2 hours after your main course, or an hour before exercising. If eaten an hour before exercising, it will ensure that these extra calories and fats are used up before they can be stored in the body. This action will also prevent excess glucose from accumulating in the body.

Drinking a glass of water with a hint of cayenne pepper prior to eating desserts will help you eat less. You will also feel fuller much faster, thus preventing overeating. If you really want to be a die-hard, add just a small pinch of cayenne pepper to your desserts. A small dash of cayenne pepper won't drown out the enormous amount of sugar contained in most desserts. However, it has been scientifically proven that cayenne pepper is very effective at preventing over consumption, helping you to feel satisfied while suppressing cravings for sweets.

6. Dining Out: These same rules apply when dining out; always have your starches and meats separately, and drink water or tea only as your primary source of hydration, and if you prefer, you may do so with a twist of lemon.

Think of each restaurant meal as not one, but two, and bring home half for tomorrow. Also, when eating Chinese food, steer clear of the fried and heavily sauced dishes, instead opting for the healthier food items on the menu.

7. Breakfast: Organic raw almonds, oatmeal, steel cut oats, and pearl barley are powerful breakfast foods and a great way to start the morning. Eating low glycemic fresh fruits just prior to or with breakfast is also highly recommended. The sweeteners of choice should be raw honey, agave nectar or stevia. A pinch of cayenne pepper is very beneficial as it will help regulate your appetite throughout the day.

8. Exercise Regularly: Perform one of the following exercises at least 3 to 4 times weekly: brisk walking, jump roping, jogging, bicycling, or swimming. (More information about this topic and the benefits associated with routine exercises are available in chapter 9.

Exercise removes toxins and stored glucose from the liver and muscles. This prepares your body to handle new glucose from your next meal. By developing and working out large muscle groups, your body will be able to burn fat and calories even while you're at rest. Make sure you get plenty of potassium to prevent muscle spasms and cramping. Eating celery, prunes, squash, oranges, and drinking grape and prune juices are all excellent sources of potassium.

9. Supplements: Everyone can benefit greatly from taking a whole food-based organic multi-vitamin, mineral, and phytonutrient supplement. Most of the foods we eat lack a great deal of vital nutrients, so the best way to compensate for this deficiency is by supplementing your regular diet.

10. Sweeteners: The majority of sugar intake should be derived from raw organic unfiltered and unprocessed sources. There are various sweeteners available like stevia (diabetic friendly), agave nectar, blackstrap molasses, raw sugar, raw honey and natural fruit.

11. Proper Meal Conception: Again, we can no longer look at the standard American diet as a model for healthy nutrition. We have been using this diet for the past 70-plus years and we have only gotten sicker and fatter. A complete meal can be whatever food you decide as long as it's healthy, properly balanced whole food.

The second point I would like to expound on is eating more than three meals per day. Because you are going to be eating properly-combined foods, you may have a desire to eat more often, and that's perfectly okay. As you lose weight and your body begins to adjust to your new eating pattern, you will naturally start eating less. As the proper ratio of friendly and hostile bacteria is restored, you will no longer crave a lot of starchy and sugary foods.

12. Meal Regularity: The more frequently you eat the less likely you are to overeat. Snacking on raw fruits and nuts can really be helpful in getting you from meal to meal without grabbing for the wrong types of foods. You can even replace some of the meats in your diet with raw nuts like almonds, walnuts, and cashews.

A report in the National Geographic magazine revealed that people who mostly consume raw nuts in place of animal meats in their diets have much lower mortality rates related to heart disease. Nuts also contain other healthier benefits that help prevent and protect against heart disease and certain cancers.

13. High Glycemic Foods: Again, if you are trying to lose weight you want to avoid combining high glycemic foods and beverages that cause a sudden rise in blood sugars (bananas, raisins, Gatorade, watermelon, popcorn, rice, potatoes, refined wheat products, ect.) with a high-fat protein (steak, fried meats, hamburgers, processed meats).

14. Whole Foods: Proper nutrition involves eating whole foods (organic if possible) containing natural fiber, minerals, and nutrients and also minimally processed. These types of food digest slower so the body doesn't get the chance to store them as fat. The fats from these sources are easily stored by the body and quickly expended by the body when needed.

Switch from eating refined products to whole grain products, and avoid over-cooking. Whole grains should normally have between 5-7 grams of fiber per serving. Although fiber is a non-caloric food, the added bulk to your meals makes you feel fuller quicker. Fiber will also collect excess fat and cholesterol, and sweep it out of the colon before it can be digested.

15. Healthy Fats: Your primary source of dietary fats should be derived from extra virgin, cold pressed olive oil. While your body cannot survive without fat, some of your daily intake of fat should solely come from olive oil and small amounts of organic flax oils. The rest can be derived from meats and nuts.

Moderate amounts of olive oil may even reduce abdominal fat if eaten as part of a diet high in plant foods. Olive oil is a mono-unsaturated fat that is easily and readily assimilated by the body. Research has shown that people who use olive as their primary source of fat have an overall balanced distribution of body fat. They actually lose weight easier than people on low-fat, high carbohydrate diets.

Also, olive oil adds lots of zest and robust flavor to your foods. Olive oil is also very beneficial for the heart, liver, and kidneys.

16. Alternative Protein: Spirulina, a plant base, blue-green algae, is high in protein containing all essential amino acids as well as vitamin B-12 and other minerals. It's the best source of plant-based protein while fish is the best source of non-plant based protein. Both are very low in fat, with spirulina containing the highest percentage of digestible protein.—

The fish of choice should be top-feeders, as they are protected by scales and living near the surface are less exposed to toxic substances. Other sources of protein are nuts, seeds, eggs, yogurt and beans. Nuts should be eaten raw only and never baked; this ensures you receive the full health benefits of their potent nutritional properties. Don't worry about the fat because they are healthy fats, which are good for you.

I eat nuts almost every day as an alternative source of meat protein. Remember to eat no more than 1 to 2oz. servings at a time. Soaking nuts overnight in hot water will also remove some of the fat for people who are less active, and it also makes then easier to digest. Sprinkle olive oil and sea salt on them after soaking and they make a great snack or main meal.

17. Meats: All meats and poultry, except for ground meats for making burgers, should be boiled first for 15 minutes to remove most of the growth hormones, antibiotics, fats, and other types of contaminants. This will also reduce the amount of fat and cholesterol in the meat itself. Boiling has always been a means of purification to remove unwanted impurities. Boiling also reduces some of the visceral fat normally packed in and around the meaty muscle parts of animal organs

Remove the skin from your poultry, as it is high in fat. You can bake or broil meats after boiling by adding a light coat of extra virgin olive oil, herbal seasonings, organic black pepper, and a tiny shake of cayenne pepper. Add sea salt in moderation and eat as much as you like along with vegetables and a big green salad. Remember, avoid eating meats with a starchy food or sweetened beverages.

18. Cayenne Pepper: Of all the herbs and spices you should have in your spice rack, cayenne pepper should be at the top of the list. In fact, if you are trying to lose weight, I recommend you replace your regular black pepper with cayenne pepper. It has been scientifically proven to help promote weight loss by helping to speed up the body's metabolism and burning excess fat. If consumed first thing in the morning is helps to regulate and suppress appetite throughout the day. Because of the heat it produces, cayenne pepper helps to transport nutrients into your cells faster as well. All it takes is a very small amount sprinkled over meals.

19. Healthy Salt: Regular table salt is unhealthy and will actually cause you to take in and retain more fluids. It is highly toxic because it only contains two minerals, sodium and chlorine, both of which are in unhealthy concentrations. It interferes with proper digestion and can cause hypertension in both sensitive and non-sodium sensitive individuals. Sea salt or Celtic sea salt is a much healthier choice.

20. Chinese Take-out: Chose dishes that feature vegetables instead of lots of meat or noodles. Ask for extra vegetables like broccoli or snow peas. Avoid deep-fried meats, seafood, or tofu, and opt for stir-fried or braised dishes. Remember to hold the heavy sauces and drink water or hot tea only if you must have a beverage with your meal. Sauces such as duck, hot mustard, hoisin, and soy should be avoided as well. Most of these portions are large enough to be shared between two people. If you are dining alone, take half the meal home for later or have it for lunch the next day. Also, if available, request brown rice instead of white rice.

21. Savor Your Food: Eat one mouthful at a time and never scarf your food down. The slower you chew and swallow your food, the healthier it is for you. Chewing food slowly also allows your body to produce the necessary hunger suppressing, satiation, and other digestive hormones that help prevent overeating.

22. Restoring Intestinal Bacteria: Improving your overall health and managing your weight is much easier when your intestinal bacteria are balanced. You can purchase a high potency pro-biotic with at least 12 billion live cultures and 12 or more different strains per capsule. You can also combine organic un-sweetened yogurt (sweeten with raw organic honey) with powdered chicory root or FOS (Fructooligosaccharides). Take this and one bulb of garlic (organic) every day for 30 days to help restore your intestinal bacteria.

23. Eat Fresh Foods: Incorporate as many fresh vegetables and fruits (except bananas, raisins, and dates) with your meals as possible. Try eating a vegetable or a combination of vegetables with lunch and dinner meals. You can also snack on fresh veggies and fruits along with raw nuts between meals. Avoid canned foods whenever possible as they are normally loaded with lots of sugar, artificial sweeteners, sodium, preservatives, and in my opinion are devoid of adequate nutrition.

24. Colon Cleanse: A healthy and active colon is the best defense against unwanted weight gain. The longer it takes for food to be processed and eliminated from the body, the more difficult it will be for you to lose weight. A colon cleanse will help rid the colon of excessive waste and reinvigorate a sluggish colon. It has been said that life and death starts in the colon. After cleaning your colon you will experience more energy as nutrients are assimilated better, allowing overall better appetite control.

25. Liver Cleanse (optional): After completing a colon cleanse, you may consider doing a liver cleanse since it is the highest fat burning organ in the body. Excessive weight stuck around the mid-section could be an indication of a liver condition known as NASH disease. Avoiding antibiotics in conjunction with a liver cleanse can help reduce the severity of this disease and may even reverse it.

26. Medications: Most Medications are toxic and often times have an ad-verse impact on the liver and kidneys. Many people gain weight when they start taking medications, and some medications used to treat diabetes like Actos and Amaryl have been proven to cause unwanted weight gain. In addition, other medications like those prescribed for hypertension and depression have also been reported to cause unwanted weight gain. It may be difficult to lose weight as rapidly as you would like to if you are taking certain medications or have taken medications over the course of many years. Whatever you do, don't stop taking your medications unless you are advised to by your doctor! As you modify your behavior, your weight will eventually become more manageable so be patient.

27. Fast Foods: When eating at your local fast food restaurants, instead of ordering the regular combo meals, order two burgers, a salad, and water instead; leave the French fries for another meal. You can also have French fries, salad, and water, and leave the burgers for another meal. Either eat, have the burger and fries separately. Remember not to drink any sweetened beverages with these types of meals.

28. Stomach Stretching and Shrinking: As food enters your stomach it begins to stretch, sending signals to your brain that you are getting full. When this happens you should start recognizing that it's time to stop eating so you don't overeat. The less often you overeat the quicker your stomach will begin to shrink to normal size. As your stomach shrinks you will naturally eat less food, which will automatically result in weight loss.

29. Fiber: Fiber helps the body burn more calories during digestion, helps you feel full longer, and triggers less fat-storing insulin than refined carbohydrates. As fiber passes through the intestines, it collects excess fat and cholesterol before it can be digested.

Fiber is bulky and non-digestible, helping to slow down digestion, which eases the absorption of glucose into the bloodstream. This unique action by fiber improves the way cells burn glucose for energy so your body will store less fat and burn more glucose. This is also important for diabetics as it helps to stabilize blood sugar levels. You can stave off hunger and reduce your overall caloric intake by consuming more fiber-rich foods with every meal. The recommended daily fiber intake is 25 to 35 grams per day.

30. Over-cooking: Avoid over-cooking starches, as this causes caramelization, which breaks down the natural fiber in whole grains. Always cook your starches slightly shorter than the time recommended in the instructions. These foods should have a stiffness-like texture and not be too soft or mushy.

31. Bitter Orange: This herb has the ability to attach and bind itself to a special subgroup of B cell receptors called B-3 receptors. This binding effect increases the rate at which fat is released from body stores for energy production, and speeds up metabolism while the body is at rest. It has replaced epinephrine in herbal weight-loss formulas.

32. Dandelion: In Europe, herbalists frequently prescribe dandelion tinctures as a weight-loss aid. Dandelion lowers water weight through its diuretic effect. It may also help the liver regulate blood sugars to avoid hypoglycemia (low blood sugar, often an immediate cause of binge eating.) Also, fat metabolism in the body increases as bile flow is stimulated by dandelion. In one laboratory study, animals that were given daily doses of dandelion extract for a month lost up to 30% of their body mass.

33. Mate: People who lose weight rapidly due to a high protein diet also lose special minerals that help keep electrolytes balanced. Mate is especially rich in minerals like magnesium, manganese, and potassium, which help the body maintain electrolyte balance caused by rapid weight loss. The primary weight-loss component of Mate is caffeine. Caffeine stimulates weight loss by short-circuiting the feedback mechanisms that keep the body from producing more adrenaline when stimulated by herbs such as ephedrine.

34. Milk Thistle: In people with Type 2 diabetes, Milk Thistle or Silymarin stimulates the liver so that it can take excess amounts of insulin out of the blood stream. Taking Silymarin as prescribed on the label counters weight gain stimulated by excessive amounts of insulin in the blood stream and by regulating the amount of insulin in circulation.

35. Wild Angelica: Insulin not only transports glucose into all cells of the body, but also transports fat into fat cells. Wild Angelica fights weight gain, which is one of the more troubling side-effects of oral medications for diabetes. Wild Angelica causes insulin to move glucose into the muscle cells rather than fat into fat cells. Certain chemicals in this herb counteract the effects of insulin, helping to prevent weight gain. By taking Wild Angelica, in conjunction with the other modifications mentioned in this book, people showing early signs of diabetes can possibly delay or prevent full-blown symptoms.

DAILY MEAL PLANNER

CHATER XII

$\mathcal{T}$his section is designed to help you learn how to eat foods in their proper combinations and proper timing. It is best to purchase organic foods whenever possible. None of the information provided here is set in stone. It is simply designed to help guide you in the direction of practicing healthier lifestyle habits. You can always incorporate your own recipe ideas as long as you stick to the nutritional principles outlined in the book.

Important Notes:

1) Start each morning by drinking 8-12 ounces of warm water or a cup of hot tea. Add a dash of cayenne pepper and sweeten to taste with (stevia, non-glycemic, and diabetic friendly {all natural herbal sweetener}or raw honey, optional). This will immediately flush your body, help suppress your appetite throughout the day, and facilitate the flow of nutrients throughout the body.

2) Since you'll be eating foods with more water content you might not have a desire to drink fluids with your meals. This is perfectly okay, you can try drinking liquids between meals if you prefer. Whenever possible do your own juicing and avoid soda and other types of sweetened beverages. If you must have something to drink with your meals, try drinking plain water or water with freshly squeezed lemon juice, or freshly brewed tea sweetened with stevia.

3) If you are short on time prepare your cooked portions in advance and refrigerate them.

4) Between meals, snack on raw nuts in moderation, or fruits and vegetables. Try to avoid all processed snack foods and dairy products (unless organic)—if you must eat them, be sure to drink lots of water with freshly squeezed lemon juice.

5) Salad dressing (½ squeezed lemon, 3 Tbsp. olive oil, 1 Tbsp. apple cider vinegar, 4oz. distilled water, Celtic Sea Salt, pepper, and non-irradiated herbal seasonings); shake well and serve.

6) All desserts, sweetened snacks, junk foods and sweetened beverages should be consumed preferably 1 hour prior to working out.

Foods to Limit or Avoid
Processed meats, canned foods, non-organic commercially processed milk, cheese and all other dairy products, refined sugar and all artificial sweeteners, table salt and salt seasonings, white flour, bleached products, fried foods, white rice, roasted nuts, commercial salad dressings, processed foods in general, junk foods, and foods that contain hydrogenated and partially hydrogenated oils, high fructose corn syrup and corn syrup based products.

Sweeteners: All refined sugar and artificial sweeteners should be immediately replaced with stevia, maple syrup, honey, blackstrap molasses, or turbinado sugar (raw sugar).

Seasoning Salts: All seasoning salts and table salts should be discarded and replaced with Celtic Sea Salt or real sea salt. Use non-irradiated Herbal Seasonings as much as possible.
It is very important that you do not overcook your meals.

Daily Detox: ½ lemon, 8 – 12 oz. cup of water, dash of cayenne pepper, maple syrup or stevia, and a pinch of Celtic Sea Salt.

Important Medical Warning: If you are diabetic consult with your doctor before implementing the program outlined below. Those who are allergic to nuts or products containing nuts can substitute with cheese if desired. The daily meal plan outlined below is a basic general guideline and can be adjusted if desired.

Monday
Breakfast: Start with fresh fruits such as melons, apples, grapes, peaches, grapefruit, oranges, ect., or raw almonds with yogurt, oatmeal, plain yogurt or boiled eggs.

Snack: Eat small serving of raw nuts (almonds, cashews, walnuts, sunflower seeds, ect., or cheese if you are allergic to nuts) with water, hot tea or freshly squeezed lemon aid.

Lunch: Spring salad, topped with chicken, herbal seasonings, nuts or beans, one or two side dishes of vegetables (optional).

Snack: fresh fruit medley (apple, orange, kiwi, grapes).

Dinner: Vegetable medley, large green salad, whole wheat bread served with one of the following; steamed brown rice, whole wheat pasta, boiled or baked potatoes.

Tuesday
Breakfast: Organic whole wheat pancakes, waffles, (Do not use commercially processed mixes or pancake syrups as they are loaded with high fructose corn syrups and other artificial sweeteners. Use your favorite naturally sweetened jam or preserve (organic if possible) or 100% pure maple syrup or raw unprocessed and unfiltered honey).

Snack: fresh fruit medley (apple, orange, kiwi, grapes).

Lunch: Baked or broiled meats or fish (salmon, tilapia, bass, perch, sardines, whiting). Meat and fish should be non-farmed raised or free range (if possible) and can be steamed as well and served with a salad and vegetables of your choice.

Snack: Cup of yogurt mixed with fresh fruit

Dinner: Baked or boiled potatoes, mixed vegetables, salad, whole wheat bread.

Wednesday

Breakfast: Organic oatmeal, whole wheat steel cut oats or organic dry cereals (soy milk (low glycemic) almond milk or rice milk.

Snack: All natural unsalted peanut butter with veggie sticks.

Lunch: Lamb chops or chicken (baked or broiled) served with spring salad and mixed vegetables.

Snack: 1/3 cup of almonds with Granny Smith apples slices.

Dinner: Wheat pasta served with marinara sauce or sautéed cabbage and sun dried tomatoes, mixed vegetables, salad, whole wheat bread.

Thursday

Breakfast: Two boiled eggs and a cup of yogurt (naturally sweetened).

Snack: fresh fruit medley (apple, orange, kiwi, grapes).

Lunch: Organic spring salad topped with cashews, almonds, sunflower seeds, walnuts and pumpkin seeds, mixed vegetables, whole wheat bread.

Snack: Eat small serving of raw nuts or cheese with water or hot tea.

Dinner: Steamed brown rice, mixed vegetables, large spring salad, whole wheat bread.

Friday

Breakfast: Whole wheat bagel with low-fat cream cheese

Snack: All natural unsalted peanut butter with veggie sticks.

Lunch: Organic spring salad, topped with tofu, mixed nuts or beans, and a side dish of vegetables.

Snack: Cup of yogurt mixed with fresh fruit

Dinner: Baked potato, mixed vegetables, large spring salad or whole wheat bread.

Saturday

Breakfast: Fresh fruit medley (melons, apples, grapes, peaches, etc.) cup of naturally sweetened yogurt.

Snack: Eat small serving of raw nuts or cheese with water or hot tea.

Lunch: Baked or broiled (salmon, Tilapia, bass, perch, sardines, whiting). Fish should be non-farm raised and can be served with salad and mixed vegetables.

Snack: fresh fruit medley (apple, orange, kiwi, grapes).

Dinner: Wheat pasta served with sautéed cabbage and sun dried tomatoes, mixed vegetables, salad, whole wheat bread.

Sunday

This is your personal day to relax and enjoy yourself. Eat whatever you want and remember to drink plenty of water and lemon with every meal and throughout the day.

ALKALIZING (WEIGHT LOSS) AND ACIDIC (WEIGHT GAIN) FOODS

CHATER XIII

Nutritional Guide

To safely lose and manage weight, your diet should consist of 80% alkaline forming foods and 20% acidic forming foods. Generally, alkaline forming foods include: most fruits, green vegetables, peas, beans, lentils, spices, herbal seasonings. Depending on which chart you look at, seeds and nuts can sometimes be labeled as both alkalizing and acidic.

Alkalizing Foods:

Alkalizing Vegetables

Alfalfa, Barley Grass, Beet Greens, Beets, Broccoli, Cabbage, Carrot, Cauliflower, Celery Chard Greens, Chlorella, Collard Greens, Cucumber, Dandelions, Dulce, Edible Flowers Eggplant, Fermented Veggie, Garlic, Green Beans, Green Peas, Kale, Kohlrabi, Lettuce, Mushrooms, Mustard Greens, Nightshade Veggies, Onions, Parsnips, Peas, Peppers, Pumpkin, Radishes, Rutabaga, Sea Veggies, Spinach, Green, Spirulina, Sprouts, Sweet Potatoes, Tomatoes, Watercress, Wheat Grass, Wild Greens.

Alkalizing Oriental Vegetables

Daikon, Dandelion Root, Kombu, Maitake, Nori, Reishi, Shiitake, Umeboshi, Wakame.

Alkalizing Fruits

Apple, Apricot, Avocado, Berries, Blackberries, Cantaloupe, Cherries, Coconut, Fresh Currants, Dates, Dried Figs, Raisins, Grapefruit, Honeydew Melon, Lemon, Lime, Muskmelons, Nectarine, Orange, Peach, Pear, Pineapple, Raisins, Raspberries, Rhubarb, Strawberries, Tangerine, Tomato, Tropical Fruits, Prunes, Watermelon.

Alkalizing Protein

Almonds (raw), Chestnuts, Millet, Tempeh (fermented), Tofu (fermented),Whey Protein Powder, Eggs (poached), Cottage Cheese, Chicken Breast, Yogurt, Chestnuts, Flax Seeds, Pumpkin Seeds, Squash Seeds, Sunflower Seeds, Millet, Sprouted Seeds.

Alkalizing Sweeteners

Stevia: 100 times sweeter than sugar, very bitter use sparingly.

Alkalizing Spices & Seasonings

Chili Pepper, Cinnamon, Curry, Ginger, Herbs (all), Miso, Mustard, Sea Salt, Tamari.

Alkalizing Other

Alkaline Antioxidant Water, Apple Cider Vinegar, Bee Pollen, Fresh Fruit Juice, Green Juices, Lecithin Granules, Mineral Water, Black strap Molasses, Probiotic Cultures, Soured Dairy Products (organic yogurt, buttermilk, etc.) Veggie Juices, Chlorella, Green Tea, Herbal Tea, Dandelion Tea, Ginseng Tea, Banchi Tea, Kombucha.

Alkalizing Minerals

Calcium: pH 12, Cesium: pH 14, Magnesium: pH 9, Potassium: pH 14, Sodium: pH 14, Although it might seem that citrus fruits would have an acidifying effect on the body, the citric acid they contain actually has an alkalinizing effect in the system.

Note: A food's acid or alkaline forming tendency in the body has nothing to do with the actual pH of the food itself before digestion. For example, lemons are very acidic; however, the end products they produce after digestion and assimilation are very alkaline, so lemons are alkaline forming in the body. Likewise, meat will test alkaline before digestion, but it leaves a very acidic residue in the body. Like nearly all animal products, meat is acid forming.

Acidic Foods:

Acidifying Vegetables

Corn, Lentils, Olives, Winter Squash.

Acidifying Fruits

Blueberries, Canned or Glazed Fruits, Cranberries, Currants, Plums, Ripe Bananas.

Acidifying Grains
Amaranth, Barley, Bran, Oat Bran, Wheat Bread, Corn, Cornstarch, Crackers, Soda, Flour, Wheat Flour, White Hemp Seed Flour, Kamut, Macaroni, Noodles, Oatmeal, Oats (rolled), Quinoa, Rice (all), Rice Cakes, Rye, Spaghetti, Spelt, Wheat Germ, Wheat.

Acidifying Beans & Legumes
Almond Milk, Black Beans, Chick Peas, Green Peas, Kidney Beans, Lentils, Pinto Beans, Red Beans, Rice Milk, Soy Beans, Soy Milk, White Beans.

Acidifying Dairy
Butter, Cheese, Ice Cream, Ice Milk.

Acidifying Nuts & Butters
Cashews, Legumes, Peanut Butter, Peanuts, Pecans, Tahini, Walnuts.

Acidifying Animal Protein
Bacon, Beef, Carp, Clams, Cod, Corned Beef, Fish, Haddock, Lamb, Lobster, Mussels, Organ Meats, Oyster, Pike, Pork, Rabbit, Salmon, Sardines, Sausage, Scallops, Shellfish, Shrimp, Tuna, Turkey, Veal, Venison.

Acidifying Fats & Oils
Avocado Oil, Butter, Canola Oil, Corn Oil, Flax Oil, Hemp Seed Oil, Lard, Olive Oil, Safflower Oil, Sesame Oil, Sunflower Oil.

Acidifying Sweeteners
Carob, Corn Syrup, Refined Sugar, Artificial Sweeteners (Aspartame, saccharin, Splenda, etc.)

Acidifying Other Foods
Catsup, Cocoa, Coffee, Mustard, Pepper, Soft Drinks, all Vinegars.

Acidifying Drugs and Chemicals
Aspirin, Chemicals, Drugs, Medicinal (all pharmaceuticals and prescriptions or over the counter), Drugs, Psychedelic Herbicides, Pesticides, Tobacco.

SOURCES

10 diets that help you lose pounds – and money. (2006). Retrieved from http://www.msnbc.msn.com/id/14604784/ns/health-diet and_nutrition/t/diets-help-you-lose-pounds---money/#.TqwY9HMdi_A

Berlin, J. A., & Coditz, G. A. (1990). A meta-analysis of physical activity in the prevention of coronary heart disease. *American Journal of Epidemiology*, 132(4), 612-628.

Big trouble in little Puerto Rico: Obese kids. (2007). Retrieved from http://www.msnbc.msn.com/id/18768818/ns/health-diet and_nutrition/t/big-trouble-little-puerto-rico-obese-kids/#.TqwYXHMdi_B

Blood pressure rising among US children: Study. (2007). Retrieved from http://www.reuters.com/article/2007/09/10/us-heart-children usa-idUSN0634417520070910

Blood pressure rising around the globe: Major risk factor not just a problem in ever-fattening Western world. (2007). Retrieved from http://www.msnbc.msn.com/id/18660422/ns/health - heart_health/t/blood-pressure-rising-around-globe/#.TqxKOXMdi_A

Bossingham, M. J., Carnell, N. S., & Campbell, W. W. (2005). Water balance, hydration status, and fat-free mass hydration in younger and older adults. *American Journal of Clinical Nutrition, 81(6), 1342-1350.*

Bouhninik, Y., Raskine, L., Simoneau, G., Paineau, D., &Bornet, F. (2006). The capacity of short-chain fructooligosaccharides to stimulate in healthy humans. *Nutrition Journal, 5, 8.*

Calle, E. E., Rodriguez, C., Walker-Thurmond, K., &Thun, M. J. (2003) Overweight, obesity, and mortality from cancer in a prospectively studied cohort of U.S. adults. *New England Journal of Medicine, 348(17), 1625-1638.*

Carroll, L. (2007). *Consumer Reports weighs in on popular diets.* Retrieved from http://www.msnbc.msn.com/id/18496858 /ns/health-diet_and_nutrition/t/consumer-reports-weighs-popular-diets/ .TqrGdnMdi_A

Chandalia, M., Garg, A., Lutjohann, D., von Bermann, K., Grungy, S. M., & Brinkley, L. J. (2000). Beneficial effects of high dietary fiber intake on patients with type 2 diabetes mellitus. *New England Journal of Medicine*, 342(19), 1392-1398.

Chinese restaurant food unhealthy, study says. (2007). Retrieved from http://www.msnbc.msn.com/id/17718517/ns/health diet_and_nutrition/t/chinese-restaurant-food-unhealthy-study-says/#.TqwZLHMdi_A

Collins, K. (2007). *French lessons: Eat petite, take your time.* Retrieved from http://www.msnbc.msn.com/id/19055377/ns/ health-diet_and_nutrition/t/french-lessons-eat-petite-take-your-time/#.TqxJc3Mdi_A

Colomer, R., & Menéndez, J. A. (2006).Mediterranean diet, olive oil and cancer. *Clinical and Translational Oncology*, 8(1), 15-21.

"Diabulimics*" skipping insulin to slim down.* (2007). Retrieved from http://www.msnbc.msn.com/id/19276475/ns/health diabetes/t/diabulimics-skipping-insulin-slim-down/#.TqpFNHMdi_A

Dieting usually fails in the long run, study finds. (2007). Retrieved from http://www.msnbc.msn.com/id/18260925/ns/health diet_and_nutrition/t/dieting-usually-fails-long-run-study-finds/#.TqxGqHMdi_A

Diet pill makers fined millions for false claims. (2007). Retrieved from http://www.msnbc.msn.com/id/16467558/ns/health

diet_and_nutrition/t/diet-pill-makers-fined-millions-false-claims/#.TqwZhXMdi_A

Diets an unhealthy fix for teen weight concerns.(2011). Retrieved from http://www.healthuponline.com/ ?p=21007

Dikeman, C. L., Murphy, M. R., &Lahey Jr., G. C. (2006). Dietary fibers affect viscosity of solutions and simulated human gastric and small intestinal digest. *The Journal of Nutrition*, 136(4), 913-919.

Dollars can motivate employees to diet. (2007). Retrieved from http://www.msnbc.msn.com/id/20960522/ns/health diet_and_nutrition/t/dollars-can-motivate-employees-diet/#.TqxHxnMdi_A

Efforts are growing to trim the fat from employees – and employers' health care costs. (2006). Retrieved from http://knowledge.wharton.upenn.edu/article.cfm?articleid=1598

Expanding waistlines add to pain at the pump: U.S. obesity linked to extra gasoline consumption, researchers say. (2006).Retrieved from http://www.msnbc.msn.com/id/15415446/ns/health-diet_and_nutrition/t/expanding-waistlines-add-pain-pump/#.TqxIVnMdi_A

Fletcher, A. (2003). *Thin for life: 10 keys to success from people who have lost weight and kept it off.* Boston, MA: Houghton Mifflin Harcourt.

Friends quit smoking? You probably will too: Smokers kick habit in groups, those who don't become outcasts, study finds. (2009). Retrieved from http://www.msnbc.msn.com/id/24759804/ns/health-addictions/t/friends-quit-smoking-you-probably-will-too/#.TqxR7nMdi_A

FTC cracks down on bogus weight-loss claims. (2004). Retrieved from http://www.msnbc.msn.com/id/6445039/ns/health-fitness/t/ftc cracks-down-bogus-weight-loss-claims/#.TqwZtHMdi_A

Gullo, S. (2004).*The thin commandments: The ten no-fail strategies for permanent weight loss*. Emmaus, PA: Rodale Books.

Harding, A. (2007). *Calories underestimated in "healthy" restaurants: Diners eat more calories than at fast food joints*. Retrieved from http://www.freerepublic.com/focus/f-news/1896603/posts

Heavy kids face hefty heart risks as they age: Rate of cardiac ills may be 16 percent higher when today's teens grow up. (2007). Retrieved from http://www.msnbc.msn.com/id/22117085/ns/health-childrens_health/t/heavy-kids-face-hefty-heart-risks-they-age/#.TqxMsXMdi_A

Herbst, R. S., Bajorin, D. F., Bleiberg, H., Blum, D., Hao, D., Johnson, B. E., Ozolos, R. F., Demetri, G. D., Ganz, P. A., Kris, M. G., Levin, B., Markman, M., Raghavan, D., Reaman, G. H., Sawaya, R., Shunchter, L. M., Sweetenham, J. W., Vahdat, L. T., Vokes, E. E., & Winn, R. J. (2006). Clinical cancer advances 2005: Major research advances in cancer treatment, prevention, and screening – A report from the American Society of Clinical Oncology. *Journal of Clinical Oncology*, 24(1), 190-205.

Institute of Medicine of the National Academies: Food and Nutrition Board. (2005). *Dietary reference intakes for energy, carbohydrate, fiber, fatty acids, cholesterol, protein, and amino acids (macronutrients)*. Washington, DC: National Academies Press.

Johnson, C. (2010). *Your muffin top may kill you: A bulging belly doubles your risk of dying within 10 years, study finds*. Retrieved from http://www.msnbc.msn.com/id/38629117/ns/health-fitness/t/your-muffin-top-may-kill-you/#.TqxG53Mdi_A

Katzmarzyk, P. T., Church, T. S., & Blair, S. N. (2004). Cardiorespiratory fitness attenuates the effects of the metabolic syndrome on all-cause and cardiovascular disease mortality in men. *Archives of Internal Medicine*, 164(10), 1092-1097.

Kay, R. M. (1982). Dietary fiber. *Journal of Lipid Research*, 23(2), 221-242.

Kuzemchak, S. (2007).*Going it alone: The do-it-yourself diet*. Retrieved from http://www.msnbc.msn.com/id/20093131/ns /health-diet_and_nutrition/t/ going-it-alone-do-it-yourself-diet/#.TqxHWnMdi_B

Lee, I. M., &Paffenbarger Jr., R. S. (2000).Association of light, moderate, and vigorous intensity physical with longevity. The Harvard Alumni Health Study. *American Journal of Epidemiology*, 151(3), 293-299.

Liechtenstein, A. H., Appel, L. J., Brands, M., Carnethon, M., Daniels, S., Franch, H. A., Franklin, B., Kris-Atherton, P., Harris, W. S., Howard, B., Karanja, N., Lefevre, M., Rudel, L., Sacks, F., Van Horn, L., Winston, M., & Wylie-Rosett, J. (2006). Diet and lifestyle recommendations revision 2006: A scientific statement from the American Heart Association Nutrition Committee. *Circulation*, 114(1), 82-96.

Malnick, S. D., & Nobler, H. (2006).The medical complications of obesity. *QJM: Monthly Journal of the Association of Physicians, 99(9)*, 565-579.

Many Britons overweight – and malnourished: Food is plentiful, but average diet is low on nutrition, experts say. (2007). Retrieved from http://www.msnbc.msn.com/id/19114067/ns/ health-diet_and_nutrition/t/many-britons-overweight-malnourished/#.TqxN5HMdi_A

Michaud, D. S., Giovannucci, E., Willett, W. C., Colditz, G. A., Stampher, M. J., & Fuchs, C. S. (2001). *Physical activity, obesity, height, and the risk of pancreatic cancer. Journal of the American Medical Association*, 286(8), 921-929.

Michels, K. B., Fuchs, C. S., Giovannucci, E., Colditz, G. A., Hunter, D. J., Stampher, M. J., & Willett, W. C. (2005) Fiber intake and incidence of colorectal cancer among 76,947 women and 74,279

men. *Cancer Epidemiology, Biomarkers, and Prevention,* 14(4),
842-849.

Most diets work about the same, study finds: People lost 10-15
pounds on programs, weight loss drugs and gained it back. (2007).
Retrieved from
http://www.msnbc.msn.com/id/19570099/#.TqxOx3Mdi_

Nomoto, K. (2005). Prevention of infections by probiotics. *Journal
of Bioscience and Bioengineering,* 100(6), 583-592.

Number of young diabetics being hospitalized increases. (2007).
Retrieved from http://forum.lowcarber.org/
showthread.php?t=359047

*Obesity rates climbed in 31 states in U.S.: Mississippi ranked No. 1
with 30 percent overweight, study found.* (2007). Retrieved from
http://www.msnbc.msn.com/id/20461564/ns/health-
diet_and_nutrition/t/obesity-rates-climbed-states-us/#.TqxO-
nMdi_A

Obesity stops jabs hitting target. (2005). Retrieved from
http://news.bbc.co.uk/2/hi/health/4477716.stm

Petersen, A. M., & Pedersen, B. K. (2005).The anti-inflammatory
effect of exercise. *Journal of Applied Physiology,* 98(4), 1154-1162.

*Poverty main cause of obesity problem in South: 50 percent in Miss.
will be heavy by 2015 if trend continues, expert says.* (2007).
Retrieved from http://www.msnbc.msn.com/id/20476824/ns/health-
diet_and_nutrition/t/poverty-main-cause-obesity-problem-
south/#.TqxPK3Mdi_A

Research may provide new link between soft drinks and weight gain.
(2005). Retrieved from http://www.biologynews.net/
archives/2005/07/31/research_may_provide_new_link_between_soft
_drinks_and_weight_gain.html

Rich-Edwards, J. W., Klienman, K., Michels, K. B., Stampher, M. J., Manson, J. E., Rexrode, K. M., Hibert, E. N., & Willet, W. C. (2005). Longitudinal study of birth weight and adult body mass index on predicting risk of coronary heart disease and stroke in women. *British Medical Journal, 330*(7500), 1115.

Rothenbacher, D., Low, M., Hardt, P. D., Klor, H. U., Ziegler, H., & Brenner, H. (2005) Prevalence and determinants of exocrine pancreatic insufficiency among older adults: Results of a population based study. *Scandinavian Journal of Gastroenterology, 40*(6), 697-704.

Sanda, B. (2004). *The double danger of high fructose corn syrup*. Retrieved from http://www.westonaprice.org/modern-foods/double-danger-of-high-fructose-corn-syrup

Scientists target soda as main cause of obesity: Nutrition experts want "fat tax" on sugar-sweetened drinks. (2006). Retrieved from http://www.msnbc.msn.com/id/11686974/ns/health-fitness/t/scientists-target-soda-main-cause-obesity/#.TqxJOHMdi_A

Silva, A. M., Wang, J., Pierson Jr., R. N., Wang, Z., Heymsfield, S. B., Sardinha, L. B., &Heshka, S. (2005). Extracellular water: Greater expansion with age in African Americans. *Journal of Applied Physiology*, 99(1), 261-267.

Soccer beats jogging for fitness, study suggests: Players had more fun, shed more fat, built more muscle and were less tired. (2007). Retrieved from http://www.msnbc.msn.com/id/20893097/ns/health-fitness/t/soccer-beats-jogging-fitness-study-suggests/#.TqxQA3Mdi_A

Stokes, M. (2008).*Why carbs are the new diet craze*. Retrieved from http://today.msnbc.msn.com/id/23189188/ns/today-today_health/t/why-carbs-are-new-diet-craze/#.TqxFinMdi_A

Taaffe, D. R. (2006).Sarcopenia—exercise as a treatment strategy. *Australian Family Physician*, 35(3), 130-134.

Teenage weight may affect later fertility. (2011). Retrieved from http://www.healthuponline.com/?p=18747

Topping, D. L., & Clifton, P. M. (2001). Short-chain fatty acids and human colonic function: Roles of resistant starch and non-starch polysaccharides. *Physiology Review, 81*(3), 1031-1064.

Tubelis, P., Stan, V., &Zachrisson, A. (2005).Increasing work-place healthiness with the probiotic lactobacillus reuteri: A randomized double-blind study in healthy humans. *Environmental Health, 4*, 25.

U.S. obesity epidemic may be leveling off: More men, kids still getting fat, but weight gain among women holds steady. (2006). Retrieved from http://www.msnbc.msn.com/id/12153886/ns/health-fitness/t/us-obesity-epidemic-may-be-leveling/#.TqxQSXMdi_A

Virtanen, K. A., Lozzo, P., Hällsten, K., Huupponen, R., Parkkola, R., Janatuinen, T., Lönnqvist, F., Viljanen, T., Ronnemaa, T., Lönnroth, P., Knuiti, J., Ferrannini, E., &Nuutila, P. (2005). Increased fat mass compensates for insulin resistance in abdominal obesity and type 2 diabetes: A position emitting tomography study. *Diabetes, 54*(9), 2720-2726.

Warburton, D. E., Nicol, C. W., &Bredin, S. S. (2006). Health benefits of physical activity: The evidence. *Canadian Medical Association Journal, 174*(6), 801-809.

Weickert, M. O., Mohlig, M., School, C., Arafat, A. M., Otto, B., Viehoff, H., Koebnick, C., Kohl, A., Spranger, J., Pfeiffer, A. F. (2006). Cereal fiber improves whole-body insulin sensitivity in overweight and obese women. *Diabetes Care, 29(4),* 775-780.

ABOUT THE AUTHOR

*J*ohn J. Finley is an entrepreneur, author, lecturer, and teacher who has touched the lives of thousands of people. He began a career in wellness over 25 years ago, but knew he had to make major self-transformations before truly pursuing his passion for helping others. Since that time, John has lost over 50 pounds, written a book about his experience, hosted his own radio show, and is a much healthier person inside and out.

John has appeared as a guest expert on over 200 radio stations across the country. Currently, he uses personal experiences and testimonials to motivate people of all ages, genders, and racial backgrounds to achieve individual health goals. In addition to individual counseling, Mr. Finley offers group classes for weight loss, nutrition, total health, fitness, and motivation. He also does seminars on all aspects of well-being for community groups, government agencies, corporations, religious organizations and public education institutions.

Mr. Finley decided to change his life almost 30 years ago. With a diagnosis of hypertension and constantly battling to control his weight, he knew it was time to do something permanent. Instead of turning to crash dieting, diet pills, and medical intervention, he chose behavior modification techniques instead.

It began simply with adding fitness to his daily routine and practicing healthier eating habits. Day by day he made small changes that ultimately led to big rewards both physically and emotionally. Four years ago, after seeing these tremendous results, Mr. Finley knew he had to utilize his knowledge and experiences to help others in the same position. He has dedicated his life to improving the lives of others through education.

With his latest book, he hopes to teach people behavior modification techniques that will inspire them to pursue healthier lifestyle habits. In addition to motivating people in wellness, John has expanded his reach to people as a personal coach. He works directly with clients to help balance all aspects of the whole life model: career, finance, physical environment, interpersonal relationships, fun/creativity, wellness, and personal development.

John provides people with a practical approach to balancing these areas. His objective is to encourage people to set goals and create action plans so they can achieve their ultimate desired state of being.